SpringerBriefs in Applied Sciences and Technology

Computational Intelligence

Series editor

Janusz Kacprzyk, Polish Academy of Sciences, Systems Research Institute, Warsaw, Poland

The series "Studies in Computational Intelligence" (SCI) publishes new developments and advances in the various areas of computational intelligence—quickly and with a high quality. The intent is to cover the theory, applications, and design methods of computational intelligence, as embedded in the fields of engineering, computer science, physics and life sciences, as well as the methodologies behind them. The series contains monographs, lecture notes and edited volumes in computational intelligence spanning the areas of neural networks, connectionist systems, genetic algorithms, evolutionary computation, artificial intelligence, cellular automata, self-organizing systems, soft computing, fuzzy systems, and hybrid intelligent systems. Of particular value to both the contributors and the readership are the short publication timeframe and the world-wide distribution, which enable both wide and rapid dissemination of research output.

More information about this series at http://www.springer.com/series/10618

Swagata Das · Devashree Tripathy
Jagdish Lal Raheja

Real-Time BCI System Design to Control Arduino Based Speed Controllable Robot Using EEG

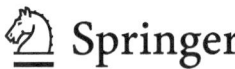 Springer

Swagata Das
Machine Vision Laboratory
CSIR-Central Electronics Engineering
Research Institute (CSIR-CEERI)
Pilani, Rajasthan, India

Jagdish Lal Raheja
Machine Vision Laboratory
CSIR-Central Electronics Engineering
Research Institute (CSIR-CEERI)
Pilani, Rajasthan, India

Devashree Tripathy
Machine Vision Laboratory
CSIR-Central Electronics Engineering
Research Institute (CSIR-CEERI)
Pilani, Rajasthan, India

ISSN 2191-530X   ISSN 2191-5318   (electronic)
SpringerBriefs in Applied Sciences and Technology
ISSN 2625-3704   ISSN 2625-3712   (electronic)
SpringerBriefs in Computational Intelligence
ISBN 978-981-13-3097-1   ISBN 978-981-13-3098-8   (eBook)
https://doi.org/10.1007/978-981-13-3098-8

Library of Congress Control Number: 2018960739

This Springer imprint is published by the registered company Springer Nature Singapore Pte Ltd.
The registered company address is: 152 Beach Road, #21-01/04 Gateway East, Singapore 189721, Singapore

Preface

Brain–computer interface (BCI) systems have always been of great use to needy paralyzed patients having the ability to provide control over any desired device. The present world calls for the need of a strong assistance system to help physically impaired people perform any anticipated task without human aid. This book proposes such a system which has the ability to perform desired actions in real time and give the impaired person a facility to move a robot in any specified direction. The system acquires the neurally impaired patient's brain signals using a SIMULINK-based model and uses their thoughts and expressions to interact with an Arduino-based speed controllable robot. It has future prospects of being implemented as a complete moving apparatus along with the patient without the involvement of any physical activity. The system is based on a graphical user interface (GUI) that will determine the direction of movement of the robot, a self-developed algorithm which preprocesses the obtained data from EMOTIV EPOC neuroheadset and then classifies the data using artificial neural network, and finally an algorithm to process the gyroscope signals using Kalman filtering to develop a mouse emulator, thereby giving the user ability to interact with the developed GUI as mentioned.

The design of mouse emulator which imitates the operations of a mouse uses the data obtained from the gyroscope embedded in the neuroheadset. The information obtained by the gyroscope in real time is used to control the relative position of the pointer which points to various operations to move the robot in the designed GUI. Hence, the proposed BCI system will perform the following primary functions:

i. The first algorithm extracts DWT coefficients from raw EEG signals and then reduces redundancy using principal component analysis (PCA). The extracted data is then used to train a neural network which has the ability to classify any preprocessed input EEG data. The dominant frequency band is generally taken under consideration for further processing.

ii. The second algorithm acquires velocity data from an embedded gyroscope. This data is then Kalman-filtered to remove unwanted jitter and noise. After conversion into displacement by integration, the final data is used to move the pointer as per the user's head movement. Thus, the user can control the mouse movement as well as click the screen whenever he/she wants to, with the help of classified data obtained from neural networks.

iii. The third part includes programming the Arduino board in order to make it capable of receiving and interpreting data successfully. The board then receives control commands from the computer to move the robot in various directions.

The above applications are integrated to control a GUI, developed in MATLAB which displays all possible movements of an Arduino-based robot. Hence, the movements of the robot can be controlled by the user by concentrating on GUI and clicking on whichever motion he/she wants. The computer communicates with the Arduino board by serial communication.

Coverage and Organization

In this section, the overview of this manuscript, which is mainly structured into five chapters, has been presented.

Chapter 1 presents a brief layout of BCI covering BCI's history, some information, BCI applications of the present and future, core concepts on BCI, and finally the objective. Chapter 2 depicts an outline of the human brain also including the fundamentals of EEG recording. Chapter 3 is a detailed portrayal of the algorithms used and to be used probably in the field of BCI. Chapter 4 is a representation of the work done in detail. Starting with the acquisition, this chapter also focuses on EEG data classification module, gyroscope signal processing, and then the final implementation of control of the robots depicting the processes of interfacing and execution.

The final Chap. 5 is a comparative overview of the complete book and the final conclusions drawn from various annotations.

Pilani, India   Swagata Das
                                                                      Devashree Tripathy
                                                                      Jagdish Lal Raheja

Contents

About the Authors

Swagata Das is pursuing her Ph.D. in biological systems engineering at Hiroshima University, Japan, having completed her M.Tech. in electronics design and technology, for which she received a gold medal at Tezpur Central University, Assam, India. She was also awarded gold medals by His Excellency Late Dr. A. P. J. Abdul Kalam, ex-President of India, and Shri. Kapil Sibal, ex-Union Minister of India, for her exceptional performance in academics at NERIST, Itanagar, India. Her research interests include electronics applications of mathematical modeling and brain–computer interface. She has published her research work in Springer and IEEE proceedings.

Devashree Tripathy completed her M.Tech. in advanced electronics systems at the CSIR-Central Electronics Engineering Research Institute. Currently, she is Ph.D. candidate in the Department of Computer Science and Engineering at the University of California, Riverside, and also Member of the SoCal Laboratory at UCR. Her research interests include computer architecture, GPGPU architecture design, high-performance computing, and fault-tolerance systems. She has worked on multiple projects on data-dependent applications on GPGPU and low-power design of GPGPU execution units and has achieved notable improvements in terms of performance gain and power and area saving. She has published papers in respected journals and conferences.

Jagdish Lal Raheja is Senior Principal Scientist and Professor at the CSIR-Central Electronics Engineering Research Institute (CSIR-CEERI). Previously, he was also Visiting Scientist at the University of Maribor, Slovenia, and Guest Scientist at the Technical University Dortmund, Germany; University College London; and the Fraunhofer-Institutszentrum Schloss Birlinghoven. His areas of specialization are image processing, pattern recognition, perception engineering, digital cartographic generalization, and artificial intelligence, and he has completed numerous research projects in these areas. He has published in various high-impact journals and conference proceedings. He is also Editorial Board Member and Reviewer for several journals and conferences.

Abbreviations

AAR	Adaptive auto regressive
AD/HD	Attention-deficit/hyperactivity disorder
ADC	Analog-to-digital converter
AIS	ASIA Impairment Scale
ASIA	American Spinal Injury Association
ALN	Adaptive logic network
ANC	Activity of neural cells
ANFIS	Adaptive neuron-fuzzy inference system
ANN	Artificial neural network
API	Application programming interface
AR	Auto regressive
BCI	Brain–computer interface
BGN	Bayesian graphical network
BLRNN	Bayesian logistic regression neural network
BMI	Brain–machine interface
BOLD	Blood oxygenation level-dependent signals
BP	Band power
CAR	Common average referencing
CGM	Conjugate gradient method
CMRR	Common mode rejection ratio
CMS	Common mode sense
CNP	Cortical neural prostheses
CNS	Central nervous system
CSPs	Common spatial patterns
CSSD	Common spatial-subspace decomposition
CSSP	Common spatio-spatial pattern
CSV	Comma-separated value
DAP	Deep anal pressure
DBI	Direct brain interface
DIL	Dual inline package

DRL	Driven right leg
DWT	Discrete wavelet transform
ECoG	Electrocorticogram
EDF	European data format
EEG	Electroencephalography
EMG	Electromyography
EML	EmoComposer Markup Language
EOG	Electrooculography
ERD	Event-related desynchronization
ERPs	Event-related potentials
ERS	Event-related synchronization
FIRNN	Finite impulse response neural network
fMRI	Functional magnetic resonance imaging
fNIRS	Functional near-infrared spectroscopy
GDNN	Gamma dynamic neural network
GMMs	Gaussian mixture models
GUI	Graphical user interface
HCI	Human Computer interface
HMM	Hidden Markov model
ICA	Independent component analysis
IDE	Integrated development environment
IOHMM	Input–output HMM
ISP	In-system programmer
kNN	k-nearest neighbors
LAT	Local averaging technique
LDA	Linear discriminant analysis
LIS	Locked-in syndrome
LVQ	Learning vector quantization
MAP	Maximum a posteriori
MLP	Multilayer perceptron
MNF	Maximum noise fraction
MNs	Multiple neuromechanisms
MRPs	Movement-related potentials
MSE	Mean square error
NIRS	Near-infrared spectroscopy
NLI	Neurological level of injury
OVR	One versus the rest
PCA	Principal component analysis
PE	Processing elements
PNS	Peripheral nervous system
PSD	Power spectral density
RBF	Radial basis function
RFLDA	Regularized Fisher's linear discriminant analysis
RMP	Resting membrane potential
ROM	Range of motion

SCG   Scaled conjugate gradient
SCP   Slow cortical potentials
SDK   Software development kit
SL   Surface Laplacian
SNR   Signal-to-noise ratio
SPS   Samples per second
SSVEP   Steady-state visual evoked potential
SVD   Singular value decomposition
SVM   Support vector machine
TCP/IP   Transmission control protocol/Internet protocol
TDNN   Time delay neural network
TTD   Thought translation device
VEPs   Visual evoked potentials
XML   Extensible Markup Language

List of Figures

List of Tables

Chapter 1
Introduction

Abstract Human–computer interfaces (HCI) are common in the present-day world. However, in situations where these are not doable, an alternate way is needed for realizing communication. This gives rise to what is also known as brain–computer interface (BCI) that provides a way of communication between the human brain and a machine in quite an effective way. BCIs are bliss for physically impaired patients. The dominant feature in a BCI is the neural activity generated in the brain by any stimulus. The concept includes encoding of brain signals through an electroencephalography (EEG) acquisition device and a computer to generate commands to gain control over another device which can be the computer cursor, a humanoid robot or an assistive mechanism. The process followed in the functionality of a BCI device can be explained as follows. It is initiated with an intent generated by the user which is meant to produce a speech, action, or motor activity. This intent, at the same time, gives rise to a complex signal with deterministic peaks in the brain, commonly known as EEG signals. The signals, when transmitted to the nervous system and to the muscles, result in performance of the intended action. The same intent generated signals when extracted through a BCI can be used to control a device helpful for the user/patient. In other words, a BCI bypasses the process of transmission of neural signals from the brain to the motor parts through a computer into an applicable device.

1.1 Brain–Computer Interface (BCI)—A Pictorial Interpretation

Ataxia is a disorder where disrupted muscle coordination affects speech, eye movement, swallowing ability, walking, picking up of objects, etc. A person affected by obstinate ataxia may have damage in the cerebellum, which is responsible for muscle coordination. The probable causes of cerebellar ataxia are a head injury, alcohol overdose, stroke, cerebral palsy, or brain tumor. Other possible situations include bleeding in the cerebellum, exposure to mercury, lead or other toxins, degenerative disorders, and head trauma. Figure 1.1 justifies the need of a brain-computer interface in different situations.

Another situation in which BCI can be beneficial is the locked-in syndrome, in which, the patient is conscious, but cannot deliberately move or talk. The patient suffers from disruption of most of the voluntary muscles. Explicit portions of the lower brain and brain stem are damaged, the upper brain being a little or not damaged. In total locked-in syndrome, the eyes are also affected by paralysis. In this case, it is very difficult for the patient to regain his/her ability to communicate or mobilize. A BCI is a very effective system that bypasses the EEG signals from the brain to another secondary device such as a wheelchair. It can be used in both the abovementioned situations, *cerebellar ataxia,* and *locked-in syndrome* (LIS). Visual feedback is a very important aspect of the operation of a BCI. For this reason, a patient suffering from total locked-in syndrome cannot use a BCI for his/her help.

1.2   History of BCI

BCIs involve numerous ideas from different fields, blended together in an intelligent manner to result in a successful process of extraction of the brain wave patterns

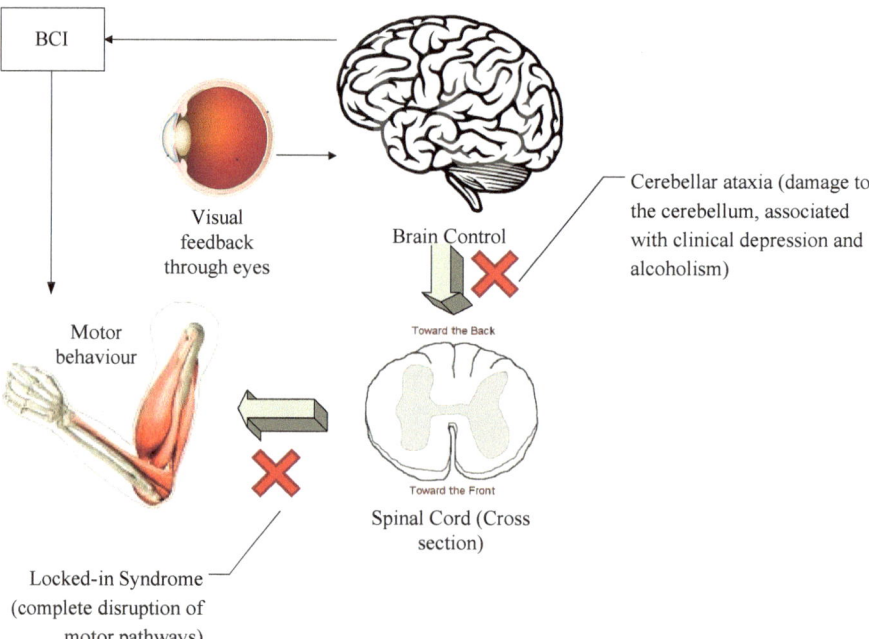

Fig. 1.1 Disruption of neural pathways as shown creates the need of a BCI which translates the EEG activity into external commands (BCI principle) (figure generated by authors)

because of external shocks and using them in a prolific way. The fields include neurosurgery, electrical engineering, computer science, and biomedical engineering all under a single umbrella (Haas 2003).

Brain research originated with Richard Canton's discovery of electrical signals on animal brain surface in 1875. EEG or electroencephalography has a major contribution in the development of BCI systems. The credit of discovery of EEG signals must be given to Hans Berger, who was responsible for the detection of brain diseases through human brain mapping in 1929 (Brain Vision UK). Another contribution to the field of BCI was of Dr. Jose Delgado for his work, in the form of a stimoceiver. Its main function was stimulation of emotions and behavior control. Dr. Delgado tested his system on a bull successfully by gaining control over its brain. This took place in the 1950s.

The first BCI designed was in the year 1964 by Dr. Grey Walter who was a neurophysiologist by profession. Dr. Walter connected electrodes to the motor areas of the brain of a patient, whose surgery was being done for some other reasons (Graimann et al. 2009). Then, the patient was asked to press a button to advance a slide projector and the corresponding brain activity was recorded. The system was then connected to a slide projector which was set to advance the slides when a similar brain activity was detected. The interesting discovery was that the system generated a button press before the patient actually pressed the button, which indicated a requirement of a delay in the system after the brainwave acquisition. Thus, a brain-controlled system was discovered and implemented for the first time. However, this work was just presented as a talk in a group called Ostler6 of a brain–computer interface based on tapping into natural electrical signals (EEG). Philip Kennedy, in 1998 implanted the first BCI into a human being. However, this device was of limited function.

BrainGate, developed by Cyberkinetics was the first commercially developed BCI in 2001 by John Donoghue and other Brown University researchers. Mathew Nagle was the first human to be implanted with the same BCI, BrainGate in Rhode Island in June 2004. In December 2004, Jonathan Wolpaw along with his group published a study depicting the ability to manipulate a computer through EEG signals picked up by a cap containing electrodes. BCI is a growing research field. It still has a lot of unexplored areas. So, let BCI expand in its scope, this work being a small contribution (Wolpaw and McFarland 2004).

1.3 More on BCI

BCIs provide an effective way for a disrupted brain to connect with the situation through a device that can interpret brain signals and convert these signals into control and command indicators. Back in the 60s, device control using brain waves was only possible in movies and was technically only a fantasy. The present situation provides enough methods to measure electrical signals out of the brain (Graimann et al. 2009). Any natural form of communication in a human being involves peripheral nervous system and muscles. The user's intent initiates the process by triggering a complex process so that certain areas of the brain are triggered. This process starts with sending signals to the concerned muscles through the peripheral nervous system, motor pathways, to be specific. Then, the concerned muscles perform the action that was indicated in the signal originated in the brain. This very action is referred to as the motor output or efferent output. The literal meaning of efferent is to convey impulses from the central to the peripheral nervous system and then to the effector or the muscle in concern. On the other hand, afferent denotes communication in the reverse direction, that is, sensory receptors to the CNS. This kind of communication is primarily important for motor skill learning and performance of agile tasks. However, the efferent pathway is essential for motion control. BCIs can be said to offer an alternate pathway to natural control and communication. It precisely sidesteps the body's regular efferent pathways.

A BCI can perform the functions of the peripheral nervous system as it directly acquires the brain activities associated with the user's intent and converts them into command signals for BCI devices. The process includes feature extraction, signal processing, and pattern recognition done within the processor of a computer. The whole system is called a brain–computer interface (BCI) as it originates from the brain activities. Following are the four important aspects to be considered while designing a BCI: The originating activities are to be recorded directly from the brain. The user must be facilitated with a real-time feedback. The system must work on intentional control of the user which means, a mental task is to be performed by the user only when he/she wants the task to be accomplished through the BCI.

BCI literature provides the following important definitions of BCI:

- "The BMI (brain machine interface) mainly aims at sending commands, originating at the cortex, which also serve as instructions or functional signals to direct the control of physically restricted body parts through machine-driven adjuncts" (Donoghue 2002).
- Through the brain computer interface, the brain is given a new type of communication which is non-muscular and enables control (Wolpaw et al. 2002).
- A brain interface uses the human brain signals to drive a machine, such as a computer or a robot and this process eliminates the need of any kind of physical movements (Levine et al. 1999).

It can be concluded that the terms brain–computer interface (BCI), brain–machine interface (BMI), and direct brain interface (DBI), all describe the same system and can be called as synonyms. Another important term, "Neuroprosthesis," is a generic term, referring to devices that can extract information from the nervous system and can also provide input by interacting with both the PNS and the CNS. BCIs are considered as a special category of neuroprostheses. Other examples of neuroprostheses are retinal implants, cochlear implants, etc.

BCI systems are often confused with mind readers. They are usually designed to recognize patterns in data extracted from the brain, which is in turn associated with commands to any secondary device. These data read from the brain are often referred to as thoughts which make BCI techniques designated as "thought-controlled." People often perceive BCIs to have the ability to tell what a person is thinking. However, the same is not true. No technical system has had this ability yet. Sensing techniques only extract brain information which is imprecise thereby representing a minuscule segment of the brain's aggregate activity. Apart from this, the total information that can be extracted from the brain can be so complex that it can barely be handled by the world's most powerful supercomputer. Another important aspect to be noted is that every brain of every individual is unique. No two persons in this world produce the same brain wave if they perform the same activity at the same time in the same environment. An important conclusion to be drawn at this point is that *"Computers cannot read anyone's mind."*

1.4 BCI Applications—Present and Future

Brain–computer interface applications are not limited to assistive care in the present-day world. Applications like gaming and other nonmedical areas have also come into the picture. Here are some common applications of today's world of brain–computer interface systems that include nonmedical areas too.

1.4.1 Communication

Communication restoration for disabled people is a top priority, especially when the person in concern is completely paralyzed or is unable to speak. The range of applications in this field is vast; covering simple binary (yes/no) abilities (Wolpaw et al. 2000), pictorial selection applications such as TalkAssist (Kennedy et al. 2000), virtual keyboards which help spell words. Keirn and Aunon (1990) created a BCI system for patients with severe physical disabilities to spell specific code words. The system could detect the difference in lateralized spectral power levels by placing electrodes all over the surface of the scalp. Farwell and Donchin (1988) developed a BCI system for typing words by making the user select letters and words from a display. They used a 6 by 6 matrix to flash letters randomly while making the user think of the next letter or word he/she wants to type. Birbaumer et al. (2000) (Perelmouter and Birbaumer 2000) give a binary speller that divides the alphabet into sequential halves until the desired letter is selected.

This speller was used by a person suffering from locked-in syndrome to compose letters in the real-world homely situation. Wolpaw et al. (2000) present a speller, slicing the alphabet into successive fourths instead of halves as in the previous. Donchin et al. (2000) have suggested a method based on the P300 component of event-related potentials. The user selects a letter by flashing rows and columns of a two-dimensional (2-D) alphabet grid to determine the desired letter. Kennedy et al. targeted locked-in subjects by providing them with a 2-D cursor navigation to select letters from a WiViK virtual keyboard (Kennedy et al. 2000). However, the spellers discussed till now could achieve an average rate of three letters per minute only, indicating a very slow rate of communication. Most of these spellers have also been used for copy spelling and free spelling. The measurement of the accuracy of the BCI output is, however, difficult and depends on user feedback.

1.4.2   Environment Control

The concept of environment control using BCI is quite helpful for improving the quality of life of severely impaired people. Such people are generally bound to stay in a closed room without much options of controlling their living environment. These types of BCIs can help them to effectively control the room's environment which may include room temperature, lighting, watching television, access to music, telephone, intelligent bed control, etc. This improvises the patient's living conditions and independence manifold. The user can operate all these devices through EEG-based BCI without any external being's help. Cincotti et al. (2008), in their work, attempted to develop a similar system and could achieve an average accuracy of 60–75%. Similar work has been done by Bayliss and Ballard (2000), where a virtual driving environment was developed to test P300 response when the subjects encountered a stoplight. The work continues with virtual interaction with virtual people and objects in a virtual apartment.

1.4.3   Movement Control with Neural Prosthesis

Another important and most researched application is the restoration of motor control in paralyzed patients. Most of these applications utilize SMR-based systems in the medical field. Such a work has been done by Wolpaw et al. that includes cursor control in all three dimensions and SMR control of a robotic arm (McFarland and Wolpaw 2008; McFarland et al. 2010; Wolpaw et al. 2002). These types of devices have helped paralyzed patients in restoring their mobility, especially by attaching orthotic devices. One such work includes Pfurtscheller et al.'s (2006) testing of SMR-based BCI for the restoration of motor control. They trained a tetraplegic (torso and limb paralyzed) patient. Recorded EEG signals over sensorimotor cortex were used to drive a hand orthosis (Pfurtscheller et al. 2000). By this orthosis, the patient could open and close his paralyzed hand successfully. Pfurtscheller et al. tested a combined system of SMR BCI with FES systems in two severe spinal injured patients.

1.4.4   Locomotion

Independent locomotion of paralyzed patients is a very important issue which can be fulfilled by BCI-based wheelchairs that can restore some form of mobility. However, in these types of applications, precision is a matter of concern. Several attempts have already been made in the development of EEG-driven wheelchairs. Some of them include Tanaka et al.'s work in (2005), Rebsamen et al.'s work of P300-BCI-based wheelchair where the user just needs to select his desired destination (Rebsamen et al. 2007). There is work still to be accomplished in this field to develop intelligent algorithms for a command system in wheelchair navigation. Accuracy is an important issue because of considerations of safety.

1.4.5 Future Expectations from BCI

Although research in this field involves signal processing and other engineering aspects only, its applications are a wide range and extend to neuroscience, engineering, psychology, neurology, and rehabilitation. The research area of BCI is still in its growing stage. Various sectors are yet to be explored which include a detailed study of accessible electrical signals of the brain, signal recording techniques, feature extraction methods, performance optimization, and increasing accuracy.

Recent work is focused on realizing laboratory setups as real-life functional home systems for the severely disabled (Vaughan et al. 2006). Such systems are currently limited to simple communication applications such as word processing, speech recognition, sending emergency messages, and simple control of home gadgets such as TV, room temperature, etc. The currently available BCI systems are not yet content because of their limited capacities, making them useful to only a small group of customers creating not much commercial interest. Other BCI applications, such as restoration of motor abilities, are still confined to research lab settings, and not yet faultless for commercialization. There is still a lot of work to be done for making BCIs validated and practically usable by homebound users.

1.5 BCI—Core Concepts

Any BCI system has common fundamental blocks of operation as given in Fig. 1.2. The first block includes the user along with acquisition device. The acquisition device helps to acquire raw EEG signals from the user's brain through electrodes. In our work, EMOTIV EPOC neuroheadset has been used as the acquisition device which comprises 14 channels along with two reference electrodes. The acquisition device also reduces noise and does initial processing of artifacts, including amplification of feeble signals. The next block is for preprocessing which does the necessary processing for bringing the raw signal up to the necessary level for further processing in the next blocks. In other words, preprocessing converts the raw data into a format which is more easily and efficiently processed by the user after this procedure.

Next, comes the feature extraction block. This block is necessary for sorting out the effective channels from the available input channels. This means feature extraction

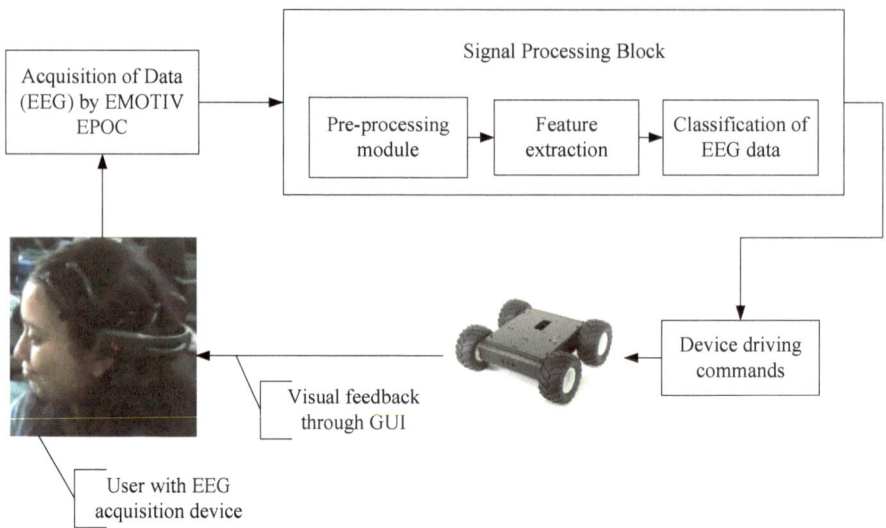

Fig. 1.2 Various blocks of BCI in the form of a block diagram (figure generated by authors; images taken from laboratory experiments)

reduces the number of input vectors for a reduced redundancy and ease of further processing. The classification block, as the name suggests, classifies the input data to provide a meaningful output which is interpretable by the user. The classified data is used by the control interface which decides the commands to be sent to the final device and provides visual feedback to the user for proper synchronization and generation of the sequential commands. The final device, as depicted in Fig. 1.2, can be a robot, a wheelchair, or a computer.

The process of brain–computer interface begins with the acquisition of raw EEG data from the user's scalp through acquisition device which also amplifies the EEG signals to a mild extent. This data is to be translated into the primary device commands, giving feedback to the user at the same time. By primary device, it means a robot or a wheelchair or any other device that the user can or wants to drive through EEG. The BCI system, thus mentioned is to be implemented in real time for proper system realization. After the acquisition of data from the user's scalp, the data are to be further processed for the consequent steps. This starts with preprocessing the acquired signals (Graimann et al. 2009). Preprocessing mainly aims at the simplification of the consequent processes without any loss of pertinent information. Upgrading the signal-to-noise ratio (SNR) of acquired signal is generally an important goal of preprocessing. The subsequent processes become easier with a better SNR. Additionally, a weaker SNR signifies that the important brain patterns are harder to detect and buried mostly in remaining part of the signal. In the step of preprocessing, unwanted signal components can be eliminated or reduced to improve the SNR.

Feature extraction is another important process following preprocessing. It primarily aims at reduction of signal dimension. Whenever the input data is too large, it tends to be more redundant. Following feature extraction, the extracted set of features (also called feature vector) is expected to contain the relevant material from raw input data. The process is called feature extraction.

Classification follows feature extraction and it becomes easier because of the preceding steps followed in the algorithm. The process of classification determines the output class that the extracted features relate to. Classification, in itself, is an algorithm. It starts with proper training by which the preprocessed and feature extracted vectors are classified as the type of data they belong to. After this, the classification algorithm is tested by running some control application and the user actions are classified using the same to determine how accurately the system works. The accuracy of the system depends on the precision of data used during system training and various other factors. Some factors include the performance of acquisition device used, user's abilities, and climatic conditions.

The most used BCI event-related potential (ERP) is the "P300 wave" which is the most easily and distinctly detectable wave in response to the stimuli (Glassman 2005; Misiti et al. 2003). Feature extraction techniques include PCA, ICA, and CSP. Similarly, classification algorithms include SVM, ANN, LDA, and some other types of pattern recognition algorithms. The classified data obtained from the algorithm is used to generate the control commands to monitor a primary device which the user is intended to drive. Another important aspect to be kept in mind is the feedback, generally in a visual, tactile, or auditory form which helps the user learn from his own actions, thereby growing his/her ability to make the overall system more and more optimized.

1.6 Objective of the Work

BCIs are of great importance as far as patient assistance is concerned. Although this field is still in its growing stage, BCIs bring up a new hope to the neurally impaired patients in regaining their motor abilities. Even though BCIs cannot provide assistance close to natural movements, they improve the living conditions of patients concerned to a pronounced extent. A BCI would not only let him interact with the environment but also drive an assistive system, such as an orthosis arm, a wheelchair or a microcomputer, as per requirement. Table 1.1 gives the score for grading muscular functionality according to the Americal Spinal Injury Association.

The user just needs to think of his intent and start his intent in his brain. The impulse generated in his brain is used to decide what the user's actual intent is and thereby is converted to a virtual action which tries to fulfill his/her desire. Prosthetic applications are also possible in future applications of BCI. However, the present situation demands mainly for BCI communication and locomotive applications. Many more applications are yet to be worked on and thought of.

In our work, the BCI designed is for driving a robot which is done in turn by a GUI using pictorial indications. The user just needs to concentrate on the GUI to

Table 1.1 Grading of muscular functions as per American Spinal Injury Association (Spinal Cord Injury Research Evidence (SCIRE): American Spinal Injury Association Impairment Scale)

Type	Description
0	Total paralysis
1	Physical or visible contraction
2	Active movement, full range of motion (ROM) with gravity eliminated
3	Active movement, full ROM against gravity
4	Active movement, full ROM against gravity, and moderate resistance in a muscle-specific position
5	(Normal) active movement, full ROM against gravity, and full resistance in a muscle-specific position expected from an otherwise unimpaired person
5*	(Normal) active movement, full ROM against gravity, and sufficient resistance to be considered normal if identified inhibiting factors (i.e., pain, disuse) were not present (Here, the asterisk '*' doesn't have any significance. It is just a measurement scale.)
NT	Not testable (i.e., due to immobilization, severe pain such that the patient cannot be graded, amputation of limbs, or contractor of >50% of the range of motion)

Table 1.2 ASIA impairment scale in detail (Spinal Cord Injury Research Evidence (SCIRE): American Spinal Injury Association Impairment Scale)

Type	Description
A	Complete. No sensory or motor function is preserved in the sacral segments S4–S5
B	Sensory incomplete. Sensory but not motor function is preserved below the neurological level and includes the sacral segments S4–S5 (light touch, pinprick at S4–S5, or deep anal pressure (DAP)), and no motor function is preserved more than three levels below the motor level on either side of the body
C	Motor incomplete. Motor function is preserved below the neurological level, and more than half of key muscle functions below the single neurological level of injury (NLI) have a muscle grade less than 3 (Grades 0–2)
D	Motor Incomplete. Motor function is preserved below the neurological level, and at least half (half or more) of key muscle functions below the NLI have a muscle grade >3
E	Normal. If sensation and motor function as tested with the ISNCSCI are graded as normal in all segments, and the patient had prior deficits, then the AIS grade is E. Someone without an initial SCI does not receive an AIS grade

select which motion he/she wants to implement. In that way, the user can drive a fully automated robot without any external help. It serves the patient with a very useful application as he/she can move the robot to any location as desired. However, the robot used is just a prototype, as future applications will involve the patient driving a wheelchair along with him/her in real time. The system is an easy realization and inexpensive at the same time.

The International Standards for Neurological Classification of Spinal Cord Injury has graded the various types of injuries at different levels (Table 1.2).

References

Bayliss, J.D., and D.H. Ballard. 2000. Recognizing evoked potentials in a virtual environment. In *Advances in Neural Information Processing Systems* 3–9.

Birbaumer, N., A. Kubler, N. Ghanayim, T. Hinterberger, J. Perelmouter, J. Kaiser, I. Iversen, B. Kotchoubey, N. Neumann, and H. Flor. 2000. The thought translation device (TTD) for completely paralyzed patients. *IEEE Transactions on Rehabilitation Engineering* 8 (2): 190–193.

Brain Vision UK. *The Brief History of Brain Computer Interfaces*. http://brainvision.co.uk/news-2/the-brief-history-of-brain-computer-interfaces-2.

Cincotti, F., D. Mattia, F. Aloise, S. Bufalari, G. Schalk, G. Oriolo, A. Cherubini, M.G. Marciani, and F. Babiloni. 2008. Non-invasive brain–computer interface system: Towards its application as assistive technology. *Brain Research Bulletin* 75 (6): 796–803.

Donchin, E., K.M. Spencer, and R. Wijesinghe. 2000. The mental prosthesis: Assessing the speed of a P300-based brain-computer interface. *IEEE Transactions on Rehabilitation Engineering* 8 (2): 174–179.

Donoghue, J.P. 2002. Connecting cortex to machines: Recent advances in brain interfaces. *Nature Neuroscience* 5: 1085–1088.

Farwell, L.A., and E. Donchin. 1988. Talking off the top of your head: Toward a mental prosthesis utilizing event-related brain potentials. *Electroencephalography and Clinical Neurophysiology* 70 (6): 510–523.

Glassman, E.L. 2005. A wavelet-like filter based on neuron action potentials for analysis of human scalp electroencephalographs. *IEEE Transactions on Biomedical Engineering* 52 (11): 1851–1862.

Grabianowski ed. *How Brain Computer Interfaces Work*. http://computer.howstuffworks.com/brain-computer-interface2.htm.

Graimann, B., B. Allison, and G. Pfurtscheller. 2009. Brain–computer interfaces: A gentle introduction. In *Brain-Computer Interfaces*, 1–27. Berlin, Heidelberg: Springer.

Haas, L.F. 2003. Hans Berger (1873–1941), Richard Caton (1842–1926), and electroencephalography. *Journal of Neurology, Neurosurgery and Psychiatry* 74 (1): 9.

Keirn, Z.A., and J.I. Aunon. 1990. A new mode of communication between man and his surroundings. *IEEE Transactions on Biomedical Engineering* 37 (12): 1209–1214.

Kennedy, P.R., R.A. Bakay, M.M. Moore, K. Adams, and J. Goldwaithe. 2000. Direct control of a computer from the human central nervous system. *IEEE Transactions on Rehabilitation Engineering* 8 (2): 198–202.

Levine, S.P., J.E. Huggins, S.L. BeMent, R.K. Kushwaha, L.A. Schuh, E.A. Passaro, M.M. Rohde, and D.A. Ross. 1999. Identification of electrocorticogram patterns as the basis for a direct brain interface. *Journal of Clinical Neurophysiology* 16 (5): 439.

McFarland, D.J., and J.R. Wolpaw. 2008. Brain-computer interface operation of robotic and prosthetic devices. *Computer* 41 (10)

McFarland, D.J., W.A. Sarnacki, and J.R. Wolpaw. 2010. Electroencephalographic (EEG) control of three-dimensional movement. *Journal of Neural Engineering* 7 (3): 036007.

Misiti, M., Y. Misiti, G. Oppenheim, and J.M. Poggi. 2003. *Les ondelettes et leurs applications*. Hermès Science Publications.

Perelmouter, J., and N. Birbaumer. 2000. A binary spelling interface with random errors. *IEEE Transactions on Rehabilitation Engineering* 8 (2): 227–232.

Pfurtscheller, G., C. Guger, G. Müller, G. Krausz, and C. Neuper. 2000. Brain oscillations control hand orthosis in a tetraplegic. *Neuroscience Letters* 292 (3): 211–214.

Pfurtscheller, G., G.R. Muller-Putz, A. Schlogl, B. Graimann, R. Scherer, R. Leeb, C. Brunner, C. Keinrath, F. Lee, G. Townsend, and C. Vidaurre. 2006. 15 years of BCI research at Graz University of Technology: Current projects. *IEEE Transactions on Neural Systems and Rehabilitation Engineering* 14 (2): 205–210.

Rebsamen, B., E. Burdet, C. Guan, H. Zhang, C.L. Teo, Q. Zeng, C. Laugier, and M.H. Ang Jr. 2007. Controlling a wheelchair indoors using thought. *IEEE Intelligent Systems*, 22 (2).

Spinal Cord Injury Research Evidence (SCIRE): American Spinal Injury Association Impairment Scale (AIS). *International Standards for Neurological Classification of Spinal Cord Injury.* http://www.scireproject.com/outcome-measures-new/american-spinal-injury-association-impairment-scale-ais-international-standards.

Tanaka, K., K. Matsunaga, and H.O. Wang. 2005. Electroencephalogram-based control of an electric wheelchair. *IEEE Transactions on Robotics* 21 (4): 762–766.

Vaughan, T.M., D.J. McFarland, G. Schalk, W.A. Sarnacki, D.J. Krusienski, E.W. Sellers, and J.R. Wolpaw. 2006. The Wadsworth BCI research and development program: at home with BCI. *IEEE Transactions on Neural Systems and Rehabilitation Engineering* 14 (2): 229–233.

Wolpaw, J.R., and D.J. McFarland. 2004. Control of a two-dimensional movement signal by a non-invasive brain-computer interface in humans. *Proceedings of the National Academy of Sciences of the United States of America* 101 (51): 17849–17854.

Wolpaw, J.R., N. Birbaumer, D.J. McFarland, G. Pfurtscheller, and T.M. Vaughan. 2002. Brain—computer interfaces for communication and control. *Clinical Neurophysiology* 113 (6): 767–791.

Wolpaw, J.R., D.J. McFarland, and T.M. Vaughan. 2000. Brain-computer interface research at the Wadsworth Center. *IEEE Transactions on Rehabilitation Engineering* 8 (2): 222–226.

Chapter 2
An Insight to the Human Brain and EEG

Abstract The human brain is a major part of the central nervous system (CNS). The CNS and the peripheral nervous system (PNS) are two major sections of the human nervous system. The CNS comprises of the brain and the spinal cord, whereas, the PNS connects the CNS to primary sensory organs of the body such as the eye, ear, nose, etc., and other organs of the body. It comprises of the spinal nerves, 12 cranial nerves, and the autonomic nerves which regulate the cardiac muscles, blood vessel wall, and gland muscles. The CNS receives information from the sensory organs and resends this information to the PNS. This chapter gives details on the human brain and its constituent features. It also discusses electroencephalography (EEG) recording, the physics behind it, EEG electrodes, their composition, and other necessary details. The last section is about the conventional EEG placement methodologies.

2.1 Neurons

Neurons can be called the basic units of the nervous system. Any cell in the nervous system has neuron as its primary component. Neurons can be of the following three types:

- Motor neurons are designated to carry data from the CNS to body organs, muscles, and glands.
- Inter-neurons act as a connecting bridge between the motor and sensory neurons.
- Sensory neurons start from receiving data from internal body organs and external stimuli and send it to the CNS, i.e., they function in reverse direction of motor neurons.

The neurons are like usual body cells in terms of their structure. The cell body is called *soma* which is essentially the largest part of the neuron. Other parts of the neuron are responsible for communication of signals from one part to another in the human body. The *axon* is responsible for carrying the signal produced by dendrites away from the cell body to other neurons. An axon can vary manifold in its length and can extend up to a meter or more. Electrical impulses are generated by the axon, also known as *action potentials*. The *axon hillock* marks the beginning of axon in the neuron and the end is usually marked by a network of branches.

An important aspect to be noted about neurons is that no two neurons are linked to each other anatomically. They are instead disconnected by very tiny physical voids that are better known as *synapses,* allowing impulses to be transmitted from one cell to another by electrical or chemical means Figs. 2.1, 2.2, 2.3 and 2.4, respectively depict the neuron, its mathematical model, the different lobes in the brain and the functional areas of the brain.

Dendrites are typical signal carriers, but in the reverse direction as compared to the axon. That is, they carry signals to the cell body. They are usually shorter in length and more branched as compared to the axon. They are the receivers of information from nearby neurons, which is why they contain many synapses.

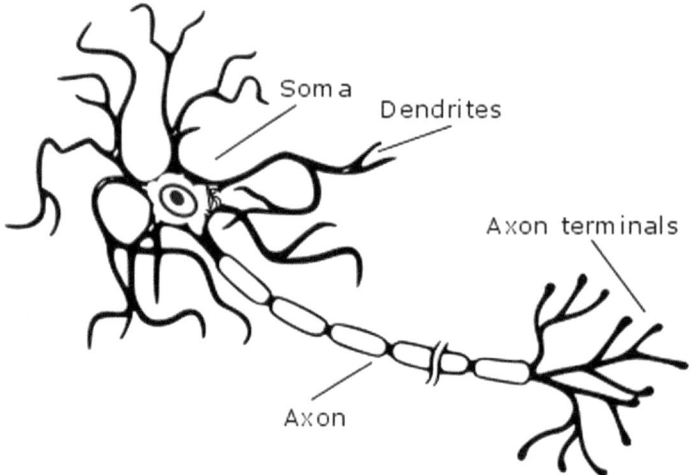

Fig. 2.1 A Typical neuron with its parts labeled (figure generated by authors)

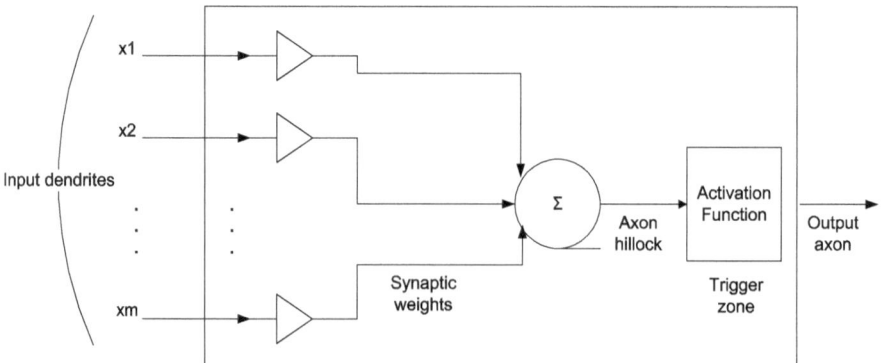

Fig. 2.2 Mathematical model of a neuron (figure generated by authors referred from Junge 1981)

Fig. 2.3 Lobes of the brain
(figure generated by authors)

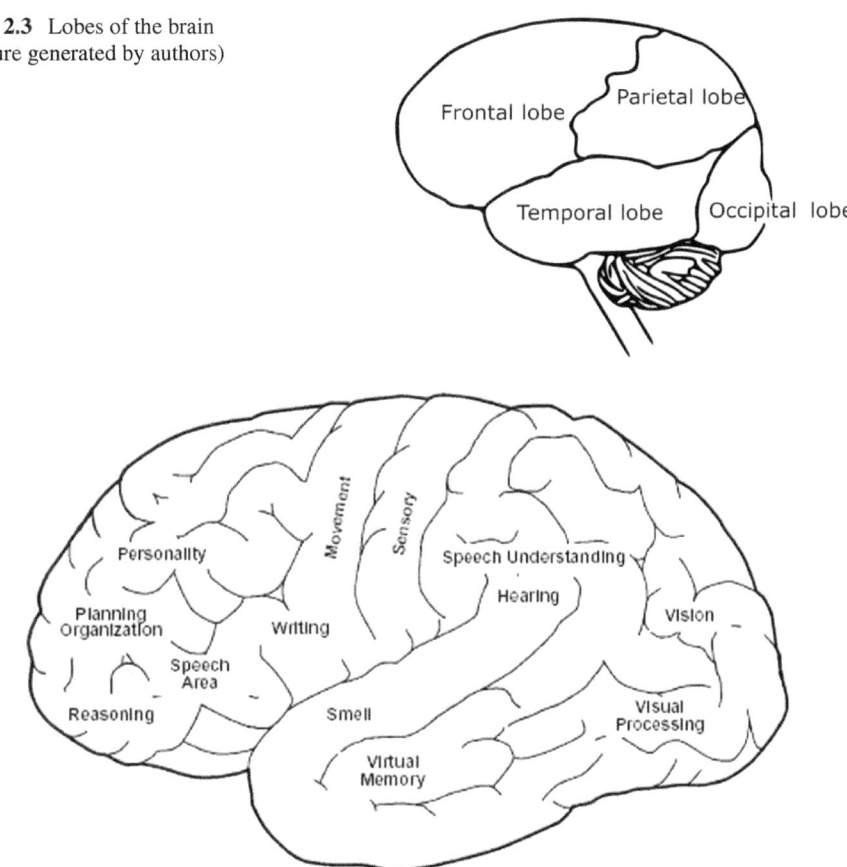

Fig. 2.4 Various functional areas of the brain in pictorial form (figure generated by authors referred from Penfield and Rasmussen 1950)

The following diagram shows a functional block diagram of a neuron which depicts how it acquires input signals through dendrites and processes those electro-chemical signals, also known as *action potentials*. The subsequent signal from the neuron is fired through the neuron's output axon. All these actions have been shown in a better way in the following diagram. It essentially analogies with a neuron concerned with the neural networks.

2.1.1 Electrical Events in Neurons

Neurons contain fluids within their thin semi-permeable membranes like other cells. All neurons are separated from the external environments by their cell membrane, also called as the plasma membrane. The membrane acts as a barrier between the intracellular and the extracellular environments of the neuron. These fluids are rich in dissolved ions, precisely, potassium and traces of sodium Na^+ and chloride Cl^- ions. These components exist in the fluid as ions, not as NaCl, salt molecule. These concentrations are just the reverse outside the cells, which means, a higher concentration of sodium Na^+ and chloride Cl^- ions and a small number of K^+ ions. The intracellular compartments are usually rich in negative ions trapped inside, making these compartments more negatively charged as compared to the extracellular compartments. An electrical voltage is generated within the nervous system by the difference in these ionic concentrations. This voltage has been mathematically represented by the Eq. 2.1 (equation of Goldman).

$$V_m = \frac{RT}{F} \ln\left(\frac{P_K[K^+]_o + P_{Na}[Na^+]_o + P_{Cl}[Cl^-]_o}{P_K[K^+]_i + P_{Na}[Na^+]_i + P_{Cl}[Cl^-]_i} \right) \approx -70 \text{ mV} \qquad (2.1)$$

where R represents the gas constant, T is the absolute temperature, and F is the Faraday's constant (Junge 1981). $[ion]_o$ and $[ion]_i$, respectively, represent the concentrations of different ions outside and inside the cell. The relative permeability of the membrane to various ions is depicted by P_K, P_{Na}, and P_{Cl}. An important aspect to be noted here is that a typical neuron at rest is said to have a membrane potential of -70 mV to -80 mV approximately, as evaluated. This can be perceived as the intracellular section being more negative than the extracellular section. In other words, the extracellular compartment is at 0 mV when the intracellular compartment is at a range of negative 70 mV to negative 80 mV during resting potential condition. This very potential is signified as the *resting membrane potential* (RMP).

It is a well-known fact that whenever ions are not externally controlled, they transport themselves through the cell membrane until a condition of equilibrium is reached, which is also known as a *chemical equilibrium*. As a result, this equilibrium has maximum chances of getting affected by any external electrical activity. Such a situation leads to nature internally controlling this external voltage by repeatedly achieving an electrical equilibrium. The *electrochemical gradient* refers to the total forces that are created by the chemical and electrical imbalances. The overall cell gradient is usually normalized by a sodium–potassium pump. K^+ ions are pumped into the cell and Na^+ ions are pumped out of the cell during the procedure, in a repeated motion whenever needed. This pump maintains the cells' signal transmitting capacity to other cells.

2.1.2   Disturbance in Equilibrium

Whenever the equilibrium of a cell is stimulated chemically, electrically or mechanically, the permeability of its membrane changes, thereby, allowing inward and outward directional flow of ions. The changes generated in the ion concentrations are directly proportional to the size of the stimulus. In this situation, the sodium–potassium pump has a major role in maintaining a concentration in the equilibrium within and outside the cell. However, in cases of high rates of flow, the pump cannot function well, resulting in a change in the resting potential (usually valued at -70 mV as mentioned).

2.1.2.1 Depolarization

The cell membrane is opened for sodium ions to flow through by a special type of protein molecules, whenever the voltage exceeds -55 mV due to a passive potential. This process is a rapid self-reinforcing cycle as it causes a further depolarization of the membrane, thereby resulting in the opening of more sodium voltage-gated channels. The process lasts for about 25 ms until all the sodium ion voltage-gated channels are opened. It is named as the *Hodgkin–Huxley Cycle*. This process of *depolarization* results in a considerable change in the membrane potential, around $+30$ mV.

2.1.2.2 Repolarization

Depolarization is followed by the opening of the membrane for potassium ions by the proteins, resulting in flowing out of potassium ions out of the cell; this process is named as *repolarization*. It marks the opening of potassium voltage-gated channels and closing of the sodium-gate channels. This process brings the membrane potential back to resting membrane potential, i.e., a negative value and is called the *absolute refractory period*. During this period, no further action potential can occur. Just after the absolute refractory period, both sodium and potassium ion voltage-gated channels remain closed for some time. This results in a further negative membrane potential. This period is called as the *relative refractory period*. The following representation depicts the overall scenario generated by an external stimulation in a neuron in terms of membrane potential.

2.2 The Human Brain

This section concentrates upon the various sections of the human brain. Sections of the human brain are primarily named as the *forebrain*, *midbrain,* and the *hindbrain*. The *cerebrum*, *thalamus*, and the *hypothalamus* comprise the forebrain. Midbrain comprises of *the tectum* and *tegmentum*. *Cerebellum*, *pons,* and the *medulla* compose the hindbrain. Often, the midbrain, pons, and medulla are together designated the name, brainstem. However, the most important part of the human brain to be focused upon in our work is the cerebral cortex as it surrounds the *cerebrum*, where most of the electrical signals are generated and emanated. The *cerebellum* is a compound part of the brain, where a majority of the thought processing and action takes place.

2.2.1 The Cerebral Cortex in More Detail

This section of the brain performs most of the important functions of the human body. It is said to be *contra-lateral* in nature. This is because the left hemisphere of the brain monitors the right side of the body and vice versa. The cerebrum comprises most of the interior of the skull. The essential count of neurons, approximately, is 100 billion in this area of the brain, each of which connects to 10 thousand other neurons making the organ a highly complicated on its own. The *cerebral cortex* holds this network altogether. Most of the functions of the human body are initiated in this part of the brain, including planning, vision, hearing, motion, sensing, and control.

It has been experimentally found that each action in concern is responsible for making changes in a definite part of the cerebrum.

The cerebral cortex is sectioned into four subsections also known as lobes:

2.2.1.1 Frontal Lobe

This is related to reasoning, planning, emotions, judgment, problem-solving, parts of speech, and motor function. In most of the right-handed people, speech is associated with the left frontal lobe located behind the forehead. Language understanding and speech are associated with the left temporal lobe located right above the ear.

2.2.1.2 Parietal Lobe

Parietal Lobe is associated with formation perception or recognition, stimuli perception, sensation, handwriting, movement, and orientation, including muscle control of the trunk, leg, arm, hand, hip, face, tongue, and vocal chords. If there is a disruption in this part of the human brain, it might create a jerk in the muscles of face or hand, sometimes, leading to one-sided paralysis of the body.

2.2.1.3 Occipital Lobe

It is at the back of the head. Occipital Lobe is mainly related to the brain's visual processing system. Distorted images could be viewed by a person if there is a disruption in this lobe, thereby making the vision appear in changed sizes.

2.2.1.4 Temporal Lobe

This is associated with memory, interpretation, and recognition of hearing stimuli. More specifically, the left section of the lobe incorporates hearing, language, and speech memory, whereas hearing and musical acknowledgment are associated with the right section.

Emotions and memory are dealt with in the deeper portions of the frontal and temporal lobes, usually called the limbic cortex. However, recent memory is related to the hippocampus, which lies just below the temporal lobe. Most of the partial seizures of the brain begin in the limbic cortex.

2.2.2   The Cortical Homunculus

The primary aim of our work is to analyze the electrical activities induced in the brain during various voluntary movements, most of which are initiated in the primary motor area. Penfield and Rasmussen (Penfield and Rasmussen 1950) in their work developed a map depicting minute areas of the primary motor area responsible for controlling different parts of the body. They have shown that the activities in specific parts of the primary motor cortex lead to motions in certain human body parts.

Cortical Homunculus is the visual depiction of the anatomical divisions in the primary motor cortex. It conceptualizes the fact that this part of the brain has "a body within the brain". In other words, any part of the human body is also present in the brain as a series of nerve structures.

It is to be noted that, the concept of homunculus mapping provides a very important clue to brain–computer interface designers as it provides important indications on the desired location of the EEG electrodes on the scalp in order to detect movement stimulated activities in the brain.

2.3   EEG Recording

This section focuses on the first step of designing a brain–computer interface system, which essentially is the extraction and recording of the electrical activities in the brain through an external device.

2.3.1   Origin

Richard Canton, in 1875, was the first individual who studied brain activities through electrodes in exposed cortexes of cats and monkeys. Since the equipment was not technically much advanced, he used galvanometers for magnification of the acquired signals and could obtain impressive results, thereby giving rise to the field of brain—computer interface. Hans Berger, a psychiatrist by profession, after 50 years, recorded the electrical activities in the brain of a human being thereby announcing the possibility of recording brain's electric activities without dissection in 1929. The same was further researched upon and named as *electroencephalogram*, EEG. It was also observed that there were variations in EEG with variations in the patient's mental state.

A major issue to be considered at this point was the origin of these brain waves. As explained earlier, most of the changes observed in EEG are initiated from the cerebral cortex. The most effective type of neuron that is responsible for generating EEG is the pyramidal cell as shown below. It can be recognized by the triangular shape of the cell body along with long parallel dendrites extending through all the layers of the cerebral cortex, usually perpendicularly placed into the surface.

2.3.2 Current Flow in Pyramidal Cell

Section 2.1.2 describes the process by which action potential is generated. A similar scenario takes place in a pyramidal cell. It starts with the triggering motion of an axon connected to a dendrite resulting the cell membrane to open up for a cluster of positively charged ions to enter. The surrounding fluid near the top of pyramid cell, resultantly, experiences a rise in the number of negative charges. Near the base of pyramid cell, an accumulation of positive charges, which initially entered the cell through the cell membrane opening, takes place. This phenomenon results in the creation of an electric dipole comprised of a pair of opposite electrical charges of equal magnitude separated by a distance. The parameters of such an electric dipole are the magnitude of its charges, $\pm q$, the separating distance, d, and the distance to the dipole, r, which are used to signify its vacuum potential given by the mathematical Eq. 2.2.

$$V_p = \frac{q\mathrm{d}.r}{4\pi\varepsilon_0|r|^3} = \frac{qd\cos\theta}{4\pi\varepsilon_0 r^2} \tag{2.2}$$

Equation 2.2 signifies an important fact, which is, the inverse relationship between the parameters, square of r and the dipole's contribution to the total electric field. This practically means, only those neurons which are very close to the electrode or directly below it, can effectively generate the EEG signal.

In addition, the direction of alignment of the pyramidal cell also plays a major role because of the cosine term in the numerator. The practical interpretation of this term is, the pyramidal cells which are perpendicular in nature to the skull can only contribute effectively to the total electric field. On the contrary, due to the presence of ridges and valleys on the magnified surface of the human brain, most of the pyramidal cells are parallel in nature, to the surface. At times, to access the perpendicular electric fields, electrodes are needed to advance inside the skull.

2.3.3   *Electrodes*

Electrodes can primarily be defined as a means by which the electrical activity in the human brain can be extracted to the input of a user-friendly recorder of EEG. Electrodes usually come in pairs, one end attached to the user's scalp and the other end to an EEG signal receiver machine. Electrodes can be of various types in case of EEG recording. Nevertheless, there is a common factor in all these kinds which is an interface of a metal and an electrolyte.

The electrode usually contains a conducting metal, whereas the electrolyte is a conducting solution. The electrical activity inside the brain is converted into a flow of electrons in the metal electrode interface layers.

2.3.3.1   Composition of Electrolyte and Electrodes

Electrolytes chosen in EEG are usually a salt solution containing sodium chloride as its principal component. This can be explained by two reasons. First, sodium chloride is highly soluble in water, which makes sodium chloride solution a rich source of sodium and chloride ions making it a very good conductor. Second, body fluids also contain these ions thus, making them compatible.

Any metal is said to be a good conductor. But to be an electrode, only some of them prove to be appropriate. When it comes in contact with the electrolyte, positive ions are released, some of which, stick to the electrode surface. Concurrently, a layer of negatively charged ions is also created in the electrolyte solution. The rates of ion layer formation differ from time to time, mostly, depending upon types of electrode and the electrolyte used. This difference in the rates of formation of ions creates another voltage at the electrode, commonly known as, the electrode potential. This is also known as half-cell potential because one electrode acts like half a battery. Recording an EEG signal always requires a pair of electrodes. That is, each one of them will have the same voltage.

Another important observation is that the pairs of electrodes must be comprised of the same material as the contrary may result in a substantial voltage between them thereby generating an unwanted artifact.

2.3.3.2   Specifications of EEG Recording Components

There are a lot of varieties of electrodes available with different characteristics. Following are the most important ones:

- **Surface electrodes**
  These consist of small metallic discs applied directly to the scalp of the patient. These discs are typically comprised of silver or gold, which barely react with the scalp. The diameter of these discs is essentially 4–10 mm ranged. A firm electrical contact is essential for fruitful results. Another important aspect to be noted here

is that a great amount of noise is created by the impedance between the electrodes and the scalp. Thus, to reduce this effect, it is vital to clean the area of concern with alcohol. For further noise reduction, certain pastes and gels can also be applied to increase the scalp conductivity and reduce the likeliness of displacement of the electrodes' position.

- **Filters**
  Most of the EEG acquisition devices contain a set of filters along with amplifiers. DC components in the signal are removed by a high-pass filter, whereas a low-pass filter removes high-frequency noise. In addition, there is also a notch filter designed to eliminate frequency components around 50/60 Hz. It reduces most of the common electrical artifacts, interference from equipment powered by alternating current.
- **Amplifiers**
  The EEG signals available from the scalp have a maximum amplitude of a few hundred microvolts. This calls for an amplifier of a very high overall gain. For this application, differential amplifiers consider a common reference for two inputs and amplify their difference. On using a differential amplifier, a major part of the noise can be eliminated.

2.3.4 Electrode Placement—The 10-20 System

The position of electrodes on the scalp define the functionality of that region of the cortex. It is also important to decide a convention of electrode placement to be able to perform tests and comparisons. In 1947, the first standard for electrode placement was developed. Following were the principles that were mutually decided:

- The positions must be such that they should be easily detectable in any subject.
- The entire human head must be considered while creating parts and naming them.
- These parts were then named according to their respective positions which were also used to name the electrodes in addition to numbers.
- The naming of the electrode should also depend upon the role of the specific section of the human brain lying under each electrode.

This convention was supervised by Herbert Jasper and was officially available in 1949 (Keirn and Aunon 1990). Named as "the 10-20 system", it is in wide use as a universal standard even after several decades.

Nasion and inion are two major points used in the electrode placement standard as shown in Fig. 2.5. The line joining these two points join the point of the brain just above the nose, and the back of the head. This line decides the electrode positions for the skull's central region. Now, there are five points which extend along this line namely, frontal pole (Fp), frontal (F), central (C), parietal (P), and occipital (O). The spacing between these points is as shown in Fig. 2.5. The name 10-20 comes from this spacing rule, which positions the electrodes at 10, 20, 20, 20, 20, and 10% of the nasion–inion distance, respectively.

Fig. 2.5 Nasion and Inion in
Brain electrode placement
(Aliki and Emmanouel 2008)

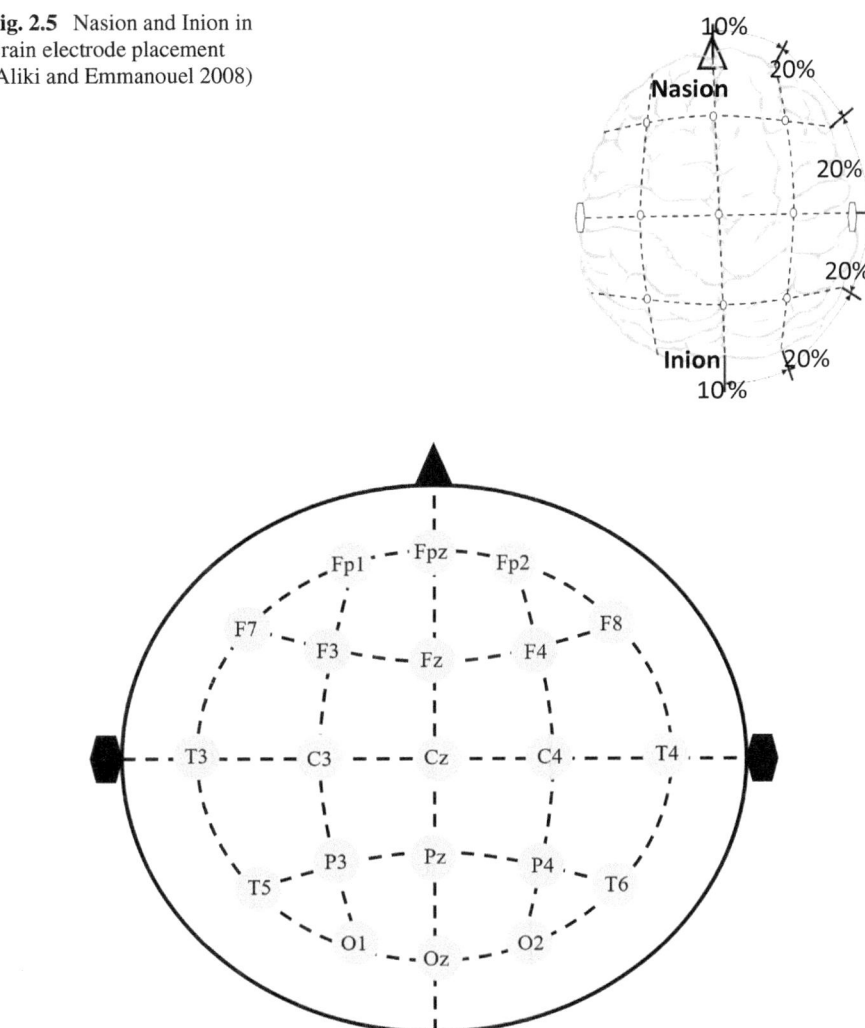

Fig. 2.6 The International 10-20 Electrode placement system (Thomas and Gaffney 2017)

The first letter of the electrode name represents its region on the skull. Apart from this, the spacing of electrodes along the horizontal line from ear to ear is done in a symmetrical manner as shown in Fig. 2.6. A similar 10-20 spacing is followed along the line extending from the forehead to the back of the head through the region above the ears. These positions are named as Fp1, F7, T3, T5, and O1 above the left ear, extending from the front to back. Along the horizontal plane, all points are equidistant. For example, Fz is equidistant to F3 and F4. Similarly, the distance between F7 and F3, F3, and Fz, Fz and F4, F4 and F8 are all same.

References

Aliki, M., and V. Emmanouel. 2008. Polysomnography: Recent Data on Procedure and Analysis, http://www.pneumon.org/assets/files/Archive/PNEUMON_2008-4.pdf#page=44.

Junge, D. 1981. *Nerve and Muscle Excitation*. 2nd ed. Sunderland, MA: Sinauer.

Keirn, Z.A., and J.I. Aunon. 1990. A new mode of communication between man and his surroundings. *IEEE Transactions on Biomedical Engineering*, 37 (12): 1209–1214.

Penfield, W., and T. Rasmussen. 1950. The cerebral cortex of man; a clinical study of localization of function.

Thomas, T.A., and A. Gaffney. 2017. Neuropsychiatric EEG—Based Assessment Aid System. *US Pharm*, 42 (1): 25–27.

Chapter 3
A Review on Algorithms for EEG-Based BCIs

Abstract Many classes of electrophysiological activities of the brain are used in designing various types of brain–computer interfaces (BCIs). Those are discussed briefly in this section. Sensorimotor activity generally corresponds to the behavior of the brain rhythms (mu, beta, and gamma), movement-related potentials (MRPs), etc. Next, the classification of BCI based on various parameters has also been discussed. These parameters are the mode of signal acquisition, timing, and placement of sensors. Later in this section, algorithms that have been and with chances of being, used in BCI applications have been discussed in a detailed manner. The algorithms chosen for each stage of the signal processing have an equal role to play in resulting a better outcome. Therefore, the section emphasizes the algorithms for each such stage, separately. Choosing a perfect algorithm is very important to design an efficient classifier. This section provides important information about the algorithms concerned with BCI.

3.1 Sensorimotor Activity

Sensorimotor cortex is the source of mu rhythms (ranging from 8 to 12 Hz) and beta rhythms (ranging from 13 to 30 Hz). These are generated when a person is not involved in sensory or motor activities. They are most distinct in the frontal and parietal lobes of the brain and make changes in the mu and lower beta bands. Any voluntary movement in the subject increases the power in the brain rhythms or frequencies. This phenomenon is also known as event-related synchronization (ERS). The peak of an ERS occurs at a delay of 600 ms following the movement offset. Finally, gamma rhythm is a high-frequency rhythm in the electroencephalography (EEG). The amplitude of gamma rhythm increases upon the occurrence of a movement.

Movement-related potentials (MRPs) usually have a maximum amplitude at the vertex with low-frequency potentials, which become more significant close to the movement. Sensorimotor activities other than the previously mentioned ones are not restricted to any particular band of frequencies or location in the brain. For example,

© The Author(s), under exclusive license to Springer Nature Singapore Pte Ltd. 2019   25
S. Das et al., *Real-Time BCI System Design to Control Arduino Based Speed Controllable Robot Using EEG*, SpringerBriefs in Computational Intelligence,
https://doi.org/10.1007/978-981-13-3098-8_3

EEG frequencies below 30 Hz may cover different event-related potentials (ERPs). However, signals of this kind do not use any specific neuromechanism.

3.1.1 Slow Cortical Potentials (SCPs)

These are steady position potentials seen in slow subjects lasting from 300 ms up to several seconds. Functionally, an SCP reflects a threshold regularization mechanism for local excitatory mobilization (Wolpaw et al. 2002).

3.1.2 P300

These waves are observable in the parietal cortex of the brain. A peak is generated at a delay of about 300 ms after stimulus reception by the brain. P300 waves are usually evoked by rare or particularly substantial visual, auditory or somatosensory stimuli when mixed with regular stimuli. The peak generated after 300 ms in said to be the P300 peak.

3.1.3 Visual Evoked Potentials (VEPs)

These are small variations produced due to visual stimuli such as a bright light. They are found to be dominant in the occipital lobe. A steady-state visual evoked potential (SSVEP) is generated when a similar stimulus continuously oscillates in front of the subject at a frequency of 5 Hz or greater. The primary difference between VEP and SSVEP is the oscillation rate of the visual stimulus.

3.1.4 Response to Mental Tasks

Various mental tasks which do not involve any nonmental task (e.g., motor activities), such as solving a mathematical question, imagining a multidimensional object, counting sheep mentally, etc., produce certain distinct distributive patterns in the EEG.

3.1.5 Activity of Neural Cells (ANC)

The activities of neural cells are highly dependent on the direction of execution of movement. The firing rates of neurons in the motor cortex increase and decrease as per the execution of movements of the neurons. Once the direction of movement is altered, the firing rate is increased or decreased accordingly.

3.1.6 Multiple Neuromechanisms (MNs)

Multiple neuromechanisms can be used by BCI systems which refer to a blend of the neuromechanisms which have been given above.

3.2 BCI-Classification

First of all, BCIs can be classified into many types according to their categories of acquisition, placement of sensors, and timing of implementation. The basic classification has been given below.

3.2.1 Classification Based on the Mode of Signal Acquisition

3.2.1.1 Online

Online means real-time implementation. Online BCI systems acquire EEG signals all the time from the user's scalp and process them in real time.

3.2.1.2 Offline

Offline analysis is performed on prerecorded data. Offline analysis can be done with already available data and can be tested for efficiency and accuracy. The implementation is not done in real time, however. So, an acquisition device is not required all the time.

3.2.2   Classification Based on Timing

3.2.2.1   Synchronous

Synchronous BCI can detect user activity automatically and take action for that reason. The user may not follow indications by the system. These systems suffer from the disadvantages of the high sensitivity of the sensors to noise. This results in a reduction of the efficiency of the algorithm to distinguish between meaningful activities and noisy signals (Graimann et al. 2009). The possibility of the user trying to connect outside time frame and trying to sit idle within the time frame is not considered. These kinds of BCIs are also named as cue-paced BCIs owing to the mode of operation. They are comparatively easy to operate and create, but the difficulty is to relate them to real-life applications. For example, it is never a good idea to make a music system which plays only at certain times or a mouse which moves the computer cursor only during limited time frames.

3.2.2.2   Asynchronous

Asynchronous BCI requires cues from the system to function. In this arrangement, the system provides the user regular cues to perform the activity. The system only responds to the activities during cue time and not otherwise. In these types of BCIs, also known as self-paced BCIs, users do not have to depend on time frames to use the BCI (Mason and Birch 2000). Terminating signals can also be sent by the user himself/herself. Therefore, asynchronous BCI or self-paced BCI analyzes brain signals of the user at all times. This mode of operation is precisely more practical and realizable to create a system that responds to the demands of the user in a highly effective and synchronized way.

3.2.3   Classification Based on the Placement of the Sensors

3.2.3.1   Non-invasive (Without Surgery)

Sensors placed on the scalp can detect activities in various sectors of the brain. When electrodes using gel base are used to acquire EEG signals, the SNR is comparatively weak (Graimann et al. 2009). Electroencephalography (EEG) denotes the recording of the electrical activities happening in the subject's brain. It is a very well-recognized method. Figure 3.1 shows a BCI making use of EEG. Advantages of EEG equipment are that they are low-budget, portable, and easier to attach. The temporal resolution of these systems is also very good. However, the disadvantages of EEG-based BCIs are that the spatial resolution and the range of operating frequency are limited. In addition to it, EEG signals are prone to get contaminated by electrical activities of

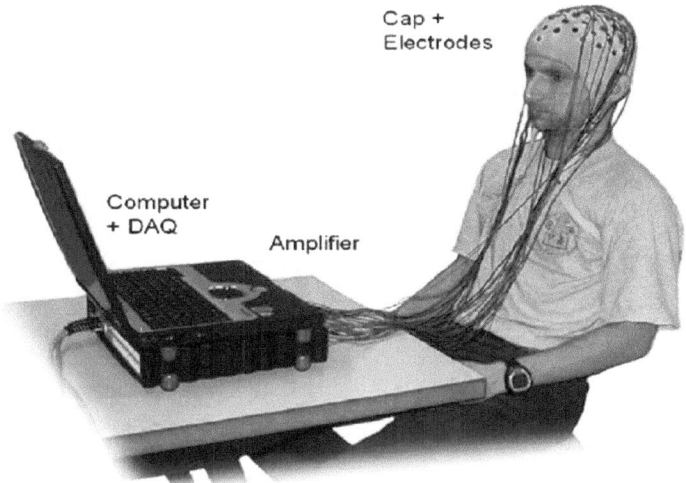

Fig. 3.1 EEG-based BCI (non-invasive) (Graimann et al. 2009)

nearby areas of the brain such as eye blinks and facial muscle movements, commonly known as electrooculographic activity (EOG) and electromyographic activity (EMG), respectively. External electromagnetic activities may also add noise to the EEG signals.

The procedure of setting up EEG becomes very tedious at times. For appropriate signal quality, proper contact of electrodes with skin is very important. Electrodes generally used are wet electrodes that use either gel or saline solutions as the medium of conduction. Wet electrodes are to be set up afresh every time they are used by the user. Dry electrodes do not have any such requirements. However, they are relatively inferior in terms of signal quality as compared to wet electrodes. As of now, scientists use the international 10–20 system of the arrangement of the electrodes over various sectors of the brain. Most BCIs use electrodes placed on the scalp. However, there are some other types of sensors too (Wolpaw et al. 2006). For example, the magnetic component of brain activities, also known as magnetoencephalography (MEG), provides useful information as well. Functional magnetic resonance imaging (fMRI) is a neuroimaging technique which measures blood flow associated with minuscule changes. The near-infrared spectroscopy (NIRS) uses the electromagnetic spectrum of 700 to 2500 nm. It can measure the optical behavior of blood with varying levels of oxygen. Researchers have experimented with the above mentioned methods by integrating them with BCI systems. However, every technique has its pros and cons. MEG and fMRI offer bulky and high-priced devices. The temporal resolution is rather poor in MEG and fMRI, and NIRS still needs to be worked on (Wolpaw et al. 2006).

Invasive (With Surgery)
Electrodes (sensors) may be placed on the skin on the scalp or can be dug into

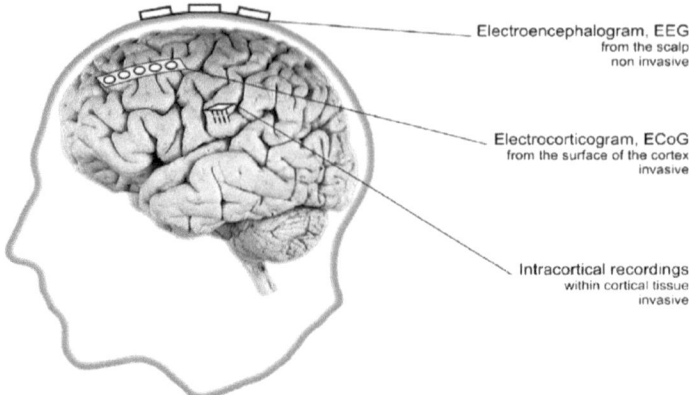

Fig. 3.2 Different BCI recording techniques (Graimann et al. 2009)

the skin. Here, sensors are implanted within the skin using surgery. A surgery called craniotomy is performed by opening the skull and making some modifications on the surface membranes. Electrocorticogram (ECoG) is the name given to such electrodes placed on the brain cortex directly. No neurons are damaged during this process as there is no involvement of penetration into the brain (Graimann et al. 2009).

Invasive recording techniques are highly advantageous with respect to (i) superior quality of the signal, (ii) excellent spatial resolution, and (iii) a higher range of operating frequencies and less problematic interferences. The need of cumbersome application and reapplication of electrodes can also be avoided. Single brain cell activity can be recorded by a process called intracortical electrodes. Invasive methods are equally disadvantageous, the most significant being the requirement of a surgery. Moral, financial and some other factors make invasive techniques very inapplicable, although brain patients who are undergoing a surgery for their treatment are comfortable with these methods.

The non-invasive BCI techniques are becoming more and more efficient with improvements in technology. However, the invasive methods are more accurate than the non-invasive methods. Figure 3.2 (Graimann et al. 2009) depicts the different BCI recordning techniques.

Another requirement in the BCI system design is a strong classification algorithm to classify the feature extracted data. Classifying the data in the form of feature vectors is a major task and of great interest in the present scenario. Such algorithms are yet being studied and evaluated for determining their critical properties and limitations (Lotte et al. 2007).

3.3 BCI Algorithms

3.3.1 Preprocessing

The processes used for the enhancement of signals prior to post/preprocessing techniques to optimize the signals for the later processes are shown below in detail. However, the choice of signal enhancement technique depends upon the technology used for capturing information and neuromechanism of the BCI system (Bashashati et al. 2007).

3.3.2 Common Average Referencing (CAR)

Spatial filters represent various methods of referencing. The location and extent of control signal determine the proper choice of a spatial filter to be used in BCI. Among all referencing methods, common average referencing (CAR) method and Laplacian method are used for BCIs that use the mu and beta ranges of brain rhythms.

3.3.3 Surface Laplacian (SL)

As already mentioned, this method is commonly used with mu and beta rhythm BCIs. There are two possible methods of Laplacian filtering namely, the large Laplacian and the small Laplacian. It has been observed that the large Laplacian method in BCI systems is comparatively superior. Another important observation made by Cincotti et al. (2003) was that a linear combination of channels implementing the Laplacian estimation was likely to have caused a highly favorable transformation of the signals to recognize different patterns in the ongoing EEG spectrum. This approved the use of only a limited number of electrodes for obtaining high recognition rates.

3.3.4 Independent Component Analysis (ICA)

ICA is an attempt to reverse the linear superposition of signals from various sources of EEG electrical potentials that project unique topography onto the "scalp maps". ICA is used to separate the EEG into components with lesser correlation. EEG signals are weighted sums of neural activities in which the path followed by the signal to reach the electrodes decide the weights. More than one electrode provides highly correlated data. If the weights are known in advance, the potentials in the sources can be computed from a sufficient number of electrode signals. ICA is a mathematical tool that solves this problem (Ungureanu et al. 2004).

3.3.5 Common Spatial Patterns (CSP)

This is the process of combination of spatially related information of EEG signals and using these combinations to enrich the final output and detect specific patterns. CSP does not need a prior selection of frequency bands for each subject. However, the discovery of these bands also provides information required for frequency-estimation and band-power methods. An important shortcoming of this method is the ample number of electrode requirement. Another major problem is the proneness to get affected by interferences. That is a single contaminated trial creates extreme changes in the filters. This can be rationalized by the achievement of a very good performance. Another shortcoming of this method is that, as it is spatial pattern based, any small change in the position of the electrodes may disrupt the classification accuracy, making it useless. The requirement for solving this problem is identical electrode position for almost every trial and every session, which is not a feasible solution, making CSP a probable failure (Ramoser et al. 2000).

3.3.6 Principal Component Analysis (PCA)

Apart from its use as a dimension reducer and a feature selector in BCIs, PCA has also been accepted as a preprocessing section in designing BCI systems. The technique focuses on the extraction of the dataset which contributes most to the variance by a linear transformation. Data that undergoes this process provides sets of lower order and higher order principal components out of which low-order components are believed to store the "rich part" of the input data. PCA is more efficient in Gaussian distributed components of data. Another important application of PCA is in classification for weighing input features, making the consecutive training process simpler and easier to execute.

Other methods of preprocessing include the following:

- Combined CSP and PCA singular value decomposition (SVD),
- Common spatio-spatial patterns (CSSP),
- Frequency normalization (Freq-Norm),
- Local averaging technique (LAT),
- Robust Kalman filtering,
- Common spatial-subspace decomposition (CSSD),
- Wiener filtering,
- Sparse component analysis,
- Maximum noise fraction (MNF),
- Spike detection methods, and
- Neuron ranking methods (ANN).

3.3.7 Classification

BCIs are aimed at translating brain activities into computer commands. This needs to be achieved either by classification or regression algorithms. The classification has been the most popular choice yet for identification of brain patterns. A BCI system is primarily based on the concept of pattern recognition. For efficient classification, it is needed to know the dominant features of BCI and the method of using them in the appropriate place. Considering time variations of EEG, BCI features are used in the most appropriate classifier. For this selection, the behavior and constraints of the features need to be clearly understood.

3.3.7.1 Feature Properties

Some of the important features associated with BCI systems include power spectral density (PSD), band powers (BP), autoregressive (AR), adaptive autoregressive (AAR) parameters, and time–frequency features. In all the features which have been attempted to work with in connection to BCIs, the following properties are significant and noteworthy:

- **Noise and outliers**: BCI features tend to contain outliers because of which, this lowers the quality of SNR in EEG signals.
- **High dimensionality**: In BCI systems, the dimensionality is usually very high. This needs to be dealt with by extraction of features from several channels and time segments and combining them intelligently.
- **Time information**: Brain activity patterns are generally linked to specific EEG variations in the time domain. Thus, BCI features contain time information.
- **Non-stationary**: EEG signals tend to vary very frequently in the time domain as well as over sessions.
- **Small training sets**: The process of collecting subjects recording training sets is a very time taking and a tedious job which results in the creation of smaller training sets.

3.3.7.2 Considering Time Variations of EEG

The patterns used to operate BCI systems are generally time-specific. In addition, these patterns have certain ranges of frequencies dominant according to the subject's status. It is vital to make use of these variations of EEG in time domain during the process of feature extraction. The following approaches are primarily used:

- **Concatenation of features from various time segments**: Features are extracted from various sections of time. These extracted features are then concatenated to form a single feature vector.

- **Combination of classifications at different time segments**: Extraction of features and classification are performed separately for various time segments. The results from these classifiers are then concatenated.
- **Dynamic classification**: In this case, a dynamic classifier is used to classify the extracted features from different time segments. The feature vectors are first used to create a temporal sequence intended to feed to the classifier.

3.3.7.3 Selection of a Classifier

The classifiers and their properties need to be analyzed before making any selection. In this section, the classifiers have been discussed in detail along with their properties. It also the issues relevant to BCI classification: (i) the curse-of-dimensionality and (ii) the bias–variance trade-off.

3.3.7.4 Classifier Categorization

There are various categories of classification for categorizing the available classifiers as per their definitions.

- **Generative–discriminative**

  Generative (or informative) classifiers (e.g., Bayes quadratic) compute the likelihood of each class and then the most probable class out of all is chosen. On the other hand, discriminative classifiers (e.g., support vector machines) are trained to classify feature vectors directly. They are trained by the way of classification.

- **Stable–unstable**

  Stable classifiers, e.g., linear discriminant analysis, are not too complex. They are relatively stable as they are not much affected by training data variations. Unstable classifiers (e.g., multilayer perceptions) are comparatively complex and more likely affected by alterations in the training data.

- **Regularized**

  Regularization means careful monitoring of the classifier's complexity. A regularized classifier is better in performing abstraction and performs well even in the presence of outliers.

- **Static–dynamic**

  Static classifiers (e.g., multilayer perceptions) classify a single feature vector. Thus, they do not use information from the temporal domain. Dynamic classifiers (e.g., hidden Markov model), on the other hand, can catch temporal dynamics which is why they can classify feature vectors in a sequential manner.

3.3.8 Problems During Classification in BCI Research

Several problems are encountered while performing classification, such as the presence of outliers, overtraining, etc. BCI associated classifiers suffer from two major problems: (i) the curse-of-dimensionality and (ii) the bias–variance trade-off (Lotte et al. 2007).

3.3.8.1 The Curse-of-Dimensionality

This means that increasing the dimensions of feature vectors results in an exponential increase in the database required to represent various classes. A small number of training sets gives poor classification results. For proper classification, the amount of training data must be prepared according to the dimensionality of the feature vectors. Unfortunately, this is not applicable in all BCI systems due to a high dimensionality and a small training set. This issue creates a major difficulty in designing BCI classifiers (Lotte et al. 2007).

3.3.8.2 The Bias–Variance Trade-Off

Classifiers usually locate the desired label y^* of a feature vector x using an f mapping. A training set T is used to develop this mapping f. However, if we consider f^* as the perfect mapping case, it remains unknown. There are three major constituents of mean square error (MSE), in terms of errors (Lotte et al. 2007):

$$\begin{aligned}
\text{MSE} &= E\left[\left(y^* - f(x)\right)^2\right] \\
&= E\left[\left(y^* - f^*(x) + f^*(x) - E[f(x)] + E[f(x)] - f(x)\right)^2\right] \\
&= E\left[\left(y^* - f^*(x)\right)^2\right] + E\left[\left(f^*(x) - E[f(x)]^2\right)\right] + E\left[\left(E[f(x)] - f(x)\right)^2\right] \\
\text{MSE} &= \text{Noise}^2 + \text{Bias}(f(x))^2 + \text{Var}(f(x)) \quad\quad\quad\quad\quad (3.1)
\end{aligned}$$

These three terms represent three types of classification error sources (Lotte et al. 2007):

- **Noise** denotes the inevitable noise inside the system.
- **Bias** represents the amount of deviation between the perfect mapping and the estimated mapping. It is mainly dependent on the technique used to obtain the mapping f.
- **Variance** denotes the errors generated from sensitivity to small fluctuations in the training set T.

The bias and variance must be both lows for a low classification error. A "natural" trade-off between bias and variance exists. A high bias and a low variance are observed in stable classifiers. On the other hand, a high variance and a low bias are seen in unstable classifiers. Simple classifiers also can perform better than complex ones. Stabilization methods are used to reduce variance. Training sets which were taken in different sessions sometimes are widely different. This issue can be solved with very low variance.

3.4   Classification Algorithms

- Linear classifiers,
- Neural networks,
- Nonlinear Bayesian classifiers,
- Nearest neighbor classifiers, and
- Combinations of classifiers.
- The most popular are briefly described and their most important properties for BCI applications are highlighted.

3.4.1   Linear Classifiers

These algorithms use linear functions to discriminate among the given data. There are two main kinds of linear classifiers that are used in BCI systems, linear discriminant analysis (LDA), and support vector machine (SVM).

3.4.2   Linear Discriminant Analysis

The LDA (also known as Fisher's LDA) method uses hyperplanes to discriminate the data into classes. For a problem with two classes, classification is relatively easier. In such cases, only a hyperplane is enough to decide which class the feature vector belongs to (Lotte et al. 2007).

The equation of the hyperplane is:

$$w_o + w^T x = 0 \quad \text{(Lotte et al. 2007)} \tag{3.2}$$

LDA uses the assumptions that the data is normally distributed and classes have the same covariance matrix. The hyperplane which separates the two classes is calculated based on the maximization of the distance between the class means and the minimization of variance between the classes. A two-class problem can be easily solved by one such plane. However, in the case of N-class problems, several of them are required. One such technique which classifies multiple class data is the "one versus the rest (OVR)" technique. This technique uses hyperplanes for separating each class from the rest. One of the advantages of this technique is low computation. This makes calculations easy, especially when used in online BCI systems. The classifier is simple and performs well too. Nevertheless, one of the major drawbacks is the linearity in the classification which makes it perform poorly for complex and nonlinear EEG data.

3.4.3 Support Vector Machine

An SVM also uses a hyperplane for the identification of classes. However, hyperplane concerning the SVM uses a different strategy. Margins are created at a distance to the nearest support vectors/training vectors and then an optimal hyperplane is decided. This process of margin maximization increases the abstraction capabilities. SVM also uses a regularization parameter C that helps to make the classifier immune to outliers and allows errors on the training set (Lotte et al. 2007).

A linear SVM is named so because it uses linear decision boundaries. This particular classifier has been applied to many synchronous BCI applications. It has been relatively more successful in the field of BCI. However, it is also possible to create nonlinear decision boundaries by raising the complexity of the classifier by the inclusion of the "kernel trick". It comprises of implicit mapping of the data to another space, using a kernel function $K(x, y)$. Gaussian or radial basis function (RBF) kernels are the generally used Kernels in BCI field (Lotte et al. 2007).

$$K(x, y) = \exp\left(\frac{-\|x - y\|^2}{2\sigma^2}\right) \tag{3.3}$$

This type has of SVMs have performed well in BCI research and also was included in multiclass pattern recognition integrated with the OVR technique. The excellent abstraction properties of SVMs and immunity to overtraining and to the curse-of-dimensionality are the major pros of SVM-based classifiers. One small drawback is the requirement of manual decisions regarding the regularization parameter C and the RBF width if the kernel is used (Lotte et al. 2007).

3.4.4 Neural Networks

Neural networks (NN) and the linear classifiers are most commonly used classifiers in the field of BCI. NN is comprised of several artificial neurons. The decision boundaries of these nets are nonlinear. The approach of most research on neural networks is the attempt to capture the precise functioning of the human brain and applying the same to computer systems. The most widely used NN for BCI is the multilayer perceptron (MLP) (Lotte et al. 2007).

3.4.4.1 Some Important Properties of Neural Networks

- **Learning property**

Learning in neural networks involves the ability to provide the desired output when fed with a definite input. The learning includes various adjustments and changes of parameters inside the network, the weights so that the finally adopted behavior matches the desired behavior as defined by the defined training dataset. The process of training is initiated by picking any example set from the training data and is fed to the network. Next, the respective output is evaluated if it matches what was expected from the target values. If it is not the desired output, the internal weights of the network are modified by following some training algorithm, so that there is a reduction in the deviation of the desired output from the actual output. In the next step, another set of training data is fed to the network and this process repeats itself until a steady state is reached and no more significant changes in the weights are required so that the system works as per the desired protocol.

- **Generalization**

Neural networks have an interesting property to generalize, that is, production of correct outputs for inputs that were not included in the training dataset of the network.

- **Nonlinearity**

In mathematical terms, NN is the mapping of an input space to an output space. The overall mapping itself can consist of smaller mappings working simultaneously in the form of simpler units called neurons. However, information processed in each neuron is in nonlinear domain resulting in the overall mapping nonlinear too. Whenever there is a physical mechanism generating the input signal, nonlinear in nature, this property of nonlinearity becomes very important.

- **Tolerance of faults**

Robust systems are meant to function normally even if parts of it are not functioning normally or stopped working, an example being the human brain. It remains unaffected even if numerous neurons die each day as a part of the natural course of events. The brain continues to work just as if nothing has happened. Performance may be altered only in conditions of severe damage to parts of it. Even in such conditions, the fall of performance is gradual in nature. It never falls suddenly to zero level to produce inappropriate outputs. This is known as *graceful degradation*. Artificial neural networks, being a lot like the human brain, also have this property of robustness.

- **Multilayer Perceptron**

An MLP consists of multiple layers of neurons: an input layer, one or more hidden layers, and an output layer. A feedforward neural network (e.g., a perceptron) uses the principle of passing the signals in a forward direction through the network. One perceptron with several inputs and single output can be called as a processing unit. The input to each neuron is connected to the output from neurons of the previous layer. On the other hand, the neurons at the output layer determine which class the input feature vector belongs to (Lotte et al. 2007).

Neural Networks and the MLP are also known as universal approximators. They have the ability to approximate any continuous function when properly trained. Additionally, several classes can also be distinguished by these classifiers. NNs are highly adaptive and flexible. MLPs tend to be very popular NNs. Many BCI-related applications use MLPs for classification. However, they can be sensitive to overtraining, when the input data is too noisy and lacks stability. When there are no hidden layers in an MLP, it is named as a perceptron (Lotte et al. 2007).

3.4.5 Nearest Neighbor Classifiers

The nearest neighbor classifiers are nonlinear yet comparatively simple classifiers. The principle of operation of these classifiers is the assignment of a feature vector to each class depending upon the location of nearest neighbor(s). These classifiers are discriminative in nature.

3.4.5.1 *k* Nearest Neighbors

The principle followed in this classification is as follows. First, the dominant class within the decision boundary is decided. This decision is taken according to the k nearest neighbors of the point whose class is to be determined. Then this class is assigned to the unknown point inside the boundary. Classification in BCI using nearest neighbor technique is commonly done by selecting the neighboring points according to their metric distance. kNN can approximate any function that can produce nonlinear decision boundaries. The only requirement is a sufficient amount of training data and a high value of k (Lotte et al. 2007).

A major drawback of kNN in BCI research is their sensitivity to the curse-of-dimensionality. However, these classifiers have performed well for BCI systems with feature vectors having low dimensionality (Lotte et al. 2007).

Figure 3.3 is an example of how kNN works. The gray spot is an unknown data which needs to be classified into one of the two classes of "stars" or "squares". Now, the value of k can be 3, 4, 5 or any other number. The smallest circle denotes the decision boundary assigned for $k = 3$. This circle has two stars and one square inside along with the unknown spot. Thus, the gray spot would be classified as a star when $k = 3$. Similarly, the bigger circle is drawn for $k = 5$. In this case, the gray spot goes with the majority, square. Similarly, for the large outer square with $k = 11$, the majority population is that of squares, due to which the spot will be classified as a square. It all depends on the intelligent decision taken to draw the boundary (Lotte et al. 2007).

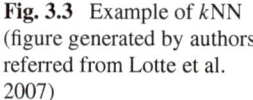

Fig. 3.3 Example of kNN (figure generated by authors referred from Lotte et al. 2007)

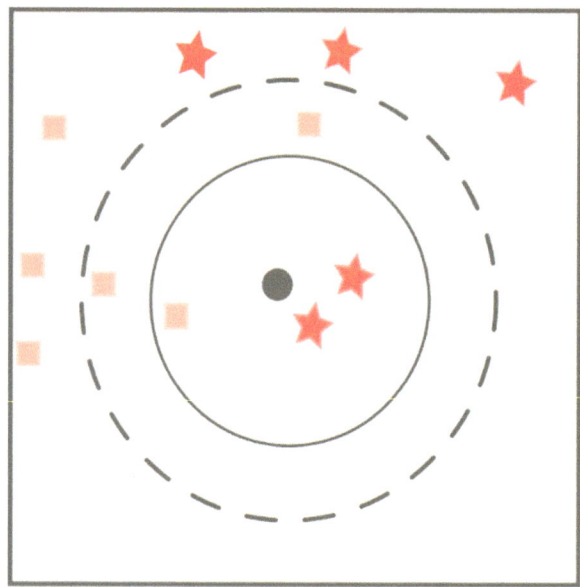

3.4.5.2 Mahalanobis Distance

In these classifiers, a Gaussian distribution, N (μ_c, M_c) is assumed for each class, c. Next, the Mahalanobis distance $d_c(x)$ is calculated, based on Eq. (3.4) (where x is the feature vector for each class) (Lotte et al. 2007):

$$d_c(x) = \sqrt{(x - \mu_c)M_c^{-1}(x - \mu_c)^{\mathrm{T}}} \tag{3.4}$$

These classifiers proved worthy for asynchronous BCI systems with multiple classes because of their robustness. However, they are still scarcely used in the real field (Lotte et al. 2007).

3.4.6 Combinations of Classifiers

In BCI-based classification, following combination strategies have been used till now:

3.4.6.1 Voting

This is a simple and efficient way of combining classifiers. The working principle is such that each type of classifier performs classification and assigns classes to each feature vector. At the end, the feature vectors are assigned that class, which gains a majority (Lotte et al. 2007).

3.4.6.2 Stacking

Multiple classifiers, known as level-0 classifiers assign classes to each input feature vector at first. Next, the output of level-0 classifiers is fed to another layer of classifiers known as meta or level-1 classifiers. The second layer of classifiers provides the final output. In the field of BCI, HMM has been used as level-0 and SVM as a level-1 classifier (Lotte et al. 2007).

The major advantage of using classifiers combinedly is their ability to outperform themselves when used individually. It has been proved that there is a reduction in variance and hence, classification error too when a combination of classifiers is used. Currently, decision tree and fuzzy classifiers have not been used yet in the BCI field.

3.4.6.3 Boosting

Each classifier in the case of boosting considers errors committed by the other classifiers. This is a step-by-step method such that the errors from the previous step are checked in the consecutive step, and so on. An intelligent classifier can be made out of weak ones by utilizing boosting technique. Unfortunately, there is a problem of mislabeling due to which it has not been applied to BCI research yet (Lotte et al. 2007).

3.5 Choosing a Perfect Classifier

The important factors under consideration for choosing a good classifier are as follows:

- Accuracy: This refers to the percentage of correct classification.
- Kappa coefficient.
- Mutual information.
- Sensitivity.
- Specificity.

The choice of a good classifier is dependent upon the type of BCI under consideration. Classifiers vary their efficiency as per their applied BCI. These differences were more evident in Synchronous and Asynchronous BCIs.

3.5.1 Synchronous BCI

Synchronous BCIs are most widely spread. The classifiers that have been proved to be efficient in these BCIs are SVMs, dynamic classifiers, and combination of classifiers.

3.5.1.1 Support Vector Machines

SVM has always given excellent results in synchronous BCIs in linear, nonlinear forms, binary, and multiclass forms. RFLDA, another classifier shares its properties with SVM. An important point to be noted here is that regularization of BCI features which are usually very noisy and likely to contain lots of outliers is a needed step. Regularized classifiers have always shown better results as compared to un-regularized, nonlinear classifiers.

SVM is also a very simple classifier that follows a kernel-spaced linear function, making it very stable and also reducing the variance. BCI features have been observed to be quite unstable in the time domain, which is why a low variance can lower the classification error to a large extent. Another point to be noted is SVM is very robust in the context of the curse-of-dimensionality. Thus, it can give satisfactory results even for high-dimensional input data and limited training sets. However, SVMs are comparatively slow classifiers, though they work fast enough with real-time BCIs.

3.5.1.2 Dynamic Classifiers

Dynamic classifiers have always outperformed static classifiers for synchronous BCIs. Feature vectors in BCIs contain temporal variations, which are probably better detected by dynamic classifiers. Dynamic classifiers have the ability to classify a sequence of low-dimensional features instead of classifying a high-dimensional feature at one time making it tough for the curse-of-dimensionality. Dynamic classifiers classify the sequence of time frames instead of just a particular time window. This way, the optimal instant for classification is not necessary to be found.

3.5.1.3 Combination of Classifiers

The combination of classifiers has always shown efficient results as compared to single classifier algorithms both in terms of accuracy and recurrence count. Preferred techniques of combination used in BCIs are Voting or Stacking. An important aspect which has been proved to be profitable by using combination techniques is the reduction of variance, which is mostly dependent on time variability, session-wise variability, or subject-wise variability (Lotte et al. 2007). Variance is mostly dependent on time variability, session-to-session variability or subject-to-subject variability. Variance is a vital source of error which can only be reduced effectively by combining classifiers as explained.

3.5.2 Asynchronous BCIs

Asynchronous BCIs have not yet been worked much upon, though dynamic classifiers do not outperform static ones in this context. Identifying the beginning of each mental task is quite a difficult job in asynchronous BCIs. This makes dynamic classifiers ineligible to use their temporal skills efficiently. Asynchronous BCIs have never used SVM and classifier combinations until now.

When it comes to synchronous BCIs, SVM is quite effective irrespective of the number of classes. Good properties of the same include simplicity, and invulnerability to the curse-of-dimensionality. The dynamic classifiers and classifier combinations are also efficient for synchronous BCIs. In the case of asynchronous BCIs, there is no comparison available as such regarding the classifiers. The following points show, which classifier can be chosen for which type of problems with BCI features:

3.5.3 Noise and Outliers

Standardized classifiers such as the SVM, tend to perform well in the presence of outliers. Systematically standardized classifiers were proposed to use in BCI systems by Muller et al. to fight outliers (Lotte et al. 2007). Discriminative classifiers are known to outperform generative classifiers in fighting outliers.

3.5.4 High Dimensionality

SVM is one of the chosen classifiers to manage feature vectors with high dimensionality. If the high dimensionality is because of a large number of time segments, dynamic classifiers can cope with the issue by working with sequences of feature vectors at a time instead of one feature vector having a high dimensionality. HMM, TDNN (dynamic classifiers), and SVMs have been found classifying BCI-related data, agreeably. During cases of low dimensionality, kNNs can also be used. Therefore, techniques of reduction of feature vector dimensionality at the root are highly suggested either by feature selection or dimensionality reduction (Lotte et al. 2007).

3.5.5   Time Information

Dynamic classifiers have the ability to efficiently use information in the temporal domain. This property makes them eligible for use in synchronous operations (Lotte et al. 2007).

3.5.6   Non-stationarity

This issue can be approached by a variance reduction technique of combination of classifiers. LDA and SVM (stable classifiers) are also applicable but combinations tend to perform way better.

3.5.7   Small Training Sets

When the training sets are small, techniques used can be relatively simple such as the LDA, that too with few parameters in demand (Lotte et al. 2007).

3.6   BCI Summary

Conventional BCIs monitor activities in the brain and then relate certain patterns with those activities. These patterns are then spotted and used to perform control and coordination. Measurement of brain activities can be done by various technologies. There are various types of BCIs including invasive and non-invasive in the first place. In addition, the brain activities are measured using multiple techniques such as electrophysiological signal capture (e.g., EEG, ECoG), NIRS, or fMRI. These techniques may also vary according to the mental strategy used to control, interface properties like mode of operation (synchronous or asynchronous), mode of feedback, the algorithm of signal processing, and type of application. Research on BCIs has been focusing on the development of control and communication technologies for sufferers of severe neuromuscular disorders and probable body paralysis or locked-in state. Assistive systems are basically aimed at by this field. They provide an effective means of control and communication for people struck by the complete locked-in syndrome.

BCIs have also possible applications for other groups of people who are less disabled, including patients of stroke, autism, and other brain disorders. The BCIs can use any form of reception including visual, sensory or proprioceptive, whichever can best recover coordination and motor abilities.

Table 3.1 Neuroheadsets: a comparative study (table generated by the authors)

Specifications	EMOTIV EPOC EEG Neuroheadset (Emotiv 2010)	Neurosky Mindwave (Signal 2015)	Xwave with Neurosky (Signal 2015)	Muse (Aimone et al. 2014)	EMOTIV INSIGHT (Emotiv 2010)
Channels	14	1 (1-ref, 1-gnd)	1 (1-ref, 1-gnd)	4	5
Sampling rate	128 Hz	512 Hz	–	220–500 Hz	128 Hz
Resolution	16-bits	12-bits	8-bits	–	–
Bandwidth	0.2–45 Hz	3–100 Hz	3–100 Hz	2–50 Hz	1–43 Hz
Dynamic range	256 mVpp	1 mVpp	–	2 mVpp	256 mVpp
Coupling mode	AC coupled	–	AC coupled	AC coupled	AC coupled
Cost	$699	$99.99	$90	$269	$299
Battery type	Li-poly	AAA	Lithium	Lithium	Li-poly
Battery life	12 h	8 h	6 h	4.5 h	4 h min run time
Remarks	Acquire four mental states, five EEG bands	Acquire two mental states	Extracts eight EEG band data	Detects positive and negative emotions, five bands of brainwaves	Captures five mental commands and six facial expressions
SDK	Yes	Yes	Yes	Yes	Yes

3.6.1 Selection of the Acquisition Device

Exploring the approachability, features, and constraints of all commercially obtainable EEG capturing headsets is very important before choosing one of them. Here, we can find a comparison of several EEG headsets including EMOTIV EEG Neuroheadset, Neurosky Mindwave Headset, Xwave with Neurosky, and the Muse Headset. The devices have upgraded themselves to a large extent in the past years in terms of cost, compactness, power requirement, battery performance, bit rate, resolution, the speed of response, quality of connectivity, efficiency, and reliability, etc. Table 3.1 denotes a comparative study of the currently available neuroheadsets referred from their respective sources (Emotiv 2010, Signal 2015 and Aimone et al. 2014).

The comparison provided above gives a true justification for why to choose the EMOTIV EPOC EEG Neuroheadset for our purpose. It provides the highest number of electrodes, user-friendly wireless interface, higher bit rate, and most importantly, a powerful battery with a long battery life.

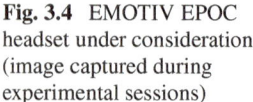
Fig. 3.4 EMOTIV EPOC
headset under consideration
(image captured during
experimental sessions)

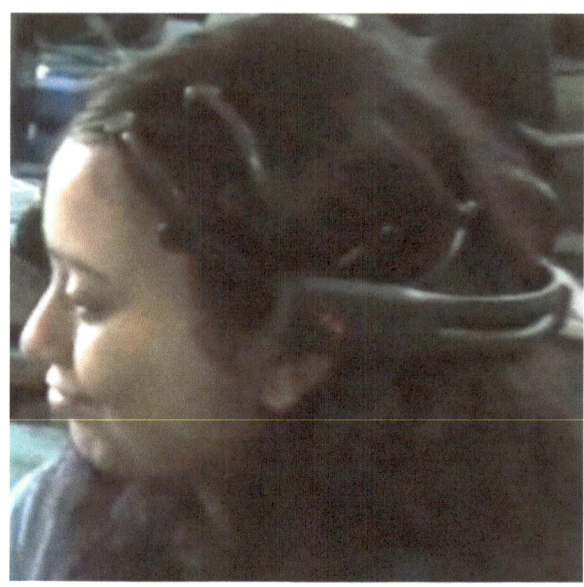

3.6.2   EMOTIV EPOC Neuroheadset

The EMOTIV EPOC EEG headset has proved itself to be the best of its kind in
the present consumer market. As compared to traditional EEG caps, this headset is
much more comfortable to wear making it more and more user-friendly. Apart from
this EPOC does not need any application of gel to the user's hair, which makes it
quite convenient and handy to use. It has only been dependent on saline electrodes
which need to be soaked in saline water before each application, much better than
applying gel on the user's hair. However, a point worth mentioning here is that getting
good quality signals in EMOTIV EPOC is a tough task on its own. It needs a lot
of patience and much processing. Before each application, the EPOC felts are to be
soaking wet in a commercially available saline solution. After applying saline to the
electrode felts, the user wears the headset on his head and signal quality is to be
checked for the purpose of calibration through the graphical user interface's visual
feedback provided by the EPOC SDK. The EPOC device communicates with the
computer through a Bluetooth dongle, the transmission being done on a proprietary
wireless band at 2.4 GHz. The user must make sure of the signal quality obtained
by looking at the graphical user interface to best for obtaining a high precision EEG
data through the headset. Figure 3.4 shows the EMOTIV EPOC headset considered
for use in this work.

  After a successful wireless connection set up by the user, the user starts obtaining
continuous EEG signals from the user's brain in real time. The data obtained from
the PC are in the form of encrypted packets using a TCP/IP socket. Depending on

the performance of the computer, it might not be possible for the network stack to pack each sample in a single TCP/IP package and send it to the SIMULINK model.

Keeping all the major aspects in mind, EMOTIV EPOC headset has been chosen as the acquisition device in our work. There are various EEG Toolboxes available in the commercial market, some of them being, FieldTrip, EEG Lab, BCILAB, LIMO EEG, BioSig, PyEEG, and OpenVIBE. However, a signal processing toolbox has been developed in this work in MATLAB after the acquisition of the raw EEG data by SIMULINK EEG Importer.

Table 3.2 shows a comparison of several EEG signal processing and analyzing toolboxes.

The SDK chosen for our purpose was the research edition SDK that cost us $750, precisely, with individual development license, including Control Panel, EmoComposer, EmoKey, TestBench, and raw EEG data API. Along with EMOTIV SDK, the EPOC SIMULINK EEG Importer was also bought costing $39.90. Through the EPOC SIMULINK EEG Importer, a MATLAB SIMULINK model can access the EEG data acquired by EMOTIV EPOC in real time. The data are received in a vector format. However, the SIMULINK environment enables it to be used for further processing. Whenever a call is made to the MATLAB MEX S-function in the SIMULINK block, it returns a vector data in the exact format as follows: COUNTER, AF3, F7, F3, FC5, T7, P7, O1, O2, P8, T8, FC6, F4, F8, AF4, GYROX, GYROY, TIMESTAMP, FUNC ID, FUNC VALUE, MARKER, and SYNC SIGNAL.

The EpocSignalServer collects EEG data samples using a TCP/IP socket to transfer the raw data to the SIMULINK S-Function. The EPOC sampling rate is 128 samples per second (SPS). Depending on the performance of the system, it might not be possible for the network stack to pack each sample in a single TCP/IP package and send it to the SIMULINK model. In the EpocSignalServer, the "samples per network package" defines the number of samples collected by the server before generating a TCP/IP message and send it to the SIMULINK model. This value can be adjusted anytime during runtime. A smaller value gives a more real-time SIMULINK model. If there is a package size of 1 sample, the SIMULINK model will run at the exact same rate as the EPOC headset (128 SPS). A smaller package size causes more frequent traffic on the network stack and there may be chances of loss of data. If such problems are encountered, the value is to be raised to a higher value on trial and error basis.

Table 3.3 gives the overall specifications of EMOTIV EPOC.

The EMOTIV EPOC EEG headset follows international 10/20 System with the modified combination nomenclature (MCN) for placement of electrodes. The MCN system renames four electrodes T3, T4, T5, and T6 as T7, T8, P7, and P8, respectively. In addition, it introduces the new positions between the previously existing points, as follows: AF—between Fp and F, FC—between F and C, FT—between F and T, CP—between C and P, TP—between T and P, PO—between P and O. Out of all 10/20 placement electrode positions, EMOTIV EPOC contains 14 electrodes along with two references called as common mode sense (CMS) and driven right leg (DRL). The CMS electrode is placed in P3 position and DRL in P4 position, thereby forming

Table 3.2 EEG toolboxes available till date (table generated by authors referred from Mahajan et al. 2014)

Toolbox	Implementation software	Objective	Features
FieldTrip	MATLAB	A flexible combination of low and high-level requirement functions. A pipeline analysis can be created by including various functions	No GUI, MATLAB functions used for user interaction-rich feature set for online and offline EEG preprocessing, ERPs, and spectral analysis
EEGLab	MATLAB	To investigate single-trial response inconsistently	Features available for performing ICA of EEG, ERPs, power spectrum, event-related, and intertrial coherence
BCILAB	MATLAB	Plugin of EEGLab, both online and offline analysis, classification of brain states using LDA and Bayesian classifier	Signal processing, feature extraction, SCPs, spectrum analysis, and nonlinear classification
PyEEG	Python	Feature vector mapping and feature extraction	21 frequency domain nonlinear features are provided
LIMOEEG	MATLAB	To analyze evoked responses over all space and time dimensions, and provide robust parametric tests	First level analysis with maximum statistics, spatial–temporal clustering-1D, 2D, ERPs, followed by second level statistical analysis
BioSig	C/C++, MATLAB/Octave	Accepting/generating signals in multiple data formats for EEG preprocessing, visualization, feature extraction, and classification	Provides vast features including time, frequency, and time–frequency transformations, common spatial pattern classification, and blind source separation
OpenVIBE	C++	Supports online signal processing and classification	Provides a platform to acquire, filter, process, and classify EEG signals

a feedback loop for referencing the other electrodes. Figure 3.5 shows a comparison of how EMOTIV EPOC adopts the international 10/20 placement.

Table 3.3 Specifications of EMOTIC EPOC (Emotiv 2010)

Number of channels	14 (plus CMS/DRL references, P3/P4 locations)
Channel names (international 10–20 locations)	AF3, F7, F3, FC5, T7, P7, O1, O2, P8, T8, FC6, F4, F8, AF4
Sampling method	Sequential sampling. Single ADC
Sampling rate	128SPS (2048 Hz internally)
Resolution	14 bits 1 LSB $= 0.51\ \mu V$ (16-bit ADC, 2 bits instrumental noise floor discarded)
Bandwidth	0.2–45 Hz, digital notch filters at 50 Hz and 60 Hz
Filtering	Built-in digital fifth-order sinc filter
Dynamic range (input referred)	8400 μV (pp)
Coupling mode	AC coupled
Power	Li-poly
Battery life (typical)	12 h
Impedance measurement	Real-time contact quality using patented system
Connectivity	Proprietary wireless, 2.4 GHz band

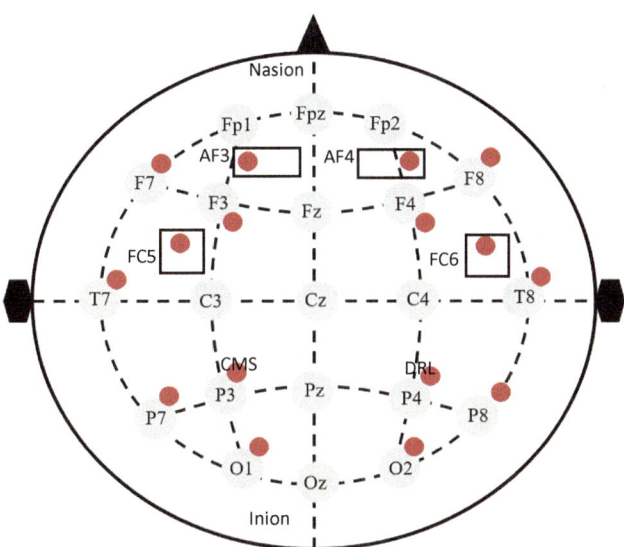

Fig. 3.5 EMOTIV electrode placement following international 10–20 placement system (Aliki and Emmanouel 2008; Emotiv 2010)

Similarly, the electrodes named AF3 and AF4 correspond to the points FP1 and FP2 in the convention. The 10/20 displacement has been shown in Fig. 3.5. The most commonly used electrodes are positioned at 10, 20, 20, 20, 20 and 10% of the path between nasion and inion points. The names given to the channels are usually same as those of the respective electrodes. That is, the signal recorded from an electrode placed at C3 would also be named as C3. The first letter usually denotes the region of the brain in concern: FP—prefrontal, AF—anterior frontal, F—frontal, C—central, P—parietal, O—occipital, T—temporal, and FC—between frontal and central lobes. The red dotted points show the electrode positions for the EMOTIV headset. The SDK provided with EMOTIV is not accessible in terms of used algorithms. No information has been provided about the technical onset of the algorithms used. However, there are some user interfaces that can be used to explore more of the EPOC and these are mentioned in this section:

3.6.2.1 Cognitiv Suite

The Cognitiv Suite records and analyzes the user's brain activities in real time. These activities are then distinguished and linked to various actions relating to a real or a virtual object (Emotiv 2010). The actions that can be detected by this suite include six directional movements (push, pull, left, right, up, and down) and six rotations (clockwise, counterclockwise, left, right, forward, and backward). In addition, another action which solely depends on the imagination power of the user is: disappear. Here, neutral actions and other actions are trained repeatedly, and this training data is segmented into short data epochs.

Using the Cognitiv Suite, any user can select up to four actions for real-time detection at one point of time. After detection, only one of those four actions is reported or else the user is found to be in a neutral state, at a particular point in time. In addition, the action power is also shown by the Cognitiv Suite relative to other actions or neutral. After the acquisition, a large number of features including spectral and other measurements are extracted followed by a feature reduction technique to classify the states in real time using the reduced feature set. Each user has a chosen set of sensors and features. If the signal quality of EEG electrodes is not good enough during a training session, then that session is discarded.

3.6.2.2 Expressiv Suite

This suite has the ability to detect various facial expressions that include blink, right/left wink, looking right/left, raise a brow, furrow brow, smile, clench, right/left smirk, and laugh. An avatar shown on the left-hand side of the Suite mimics the facial expressions of the user. On the right-hand side of the panel, sensitivity and training panels can be found. Sensitivity slider increases or decreases the speed of response of the EPOC for a particular expression. Training panel can be used to train the system for a particular expression explicitly. The various expressions that can be detected by the panel are as follows:

- **Blink**: When high, it indicates the occurrence of a blink.
- **Right Wink/Left Wink**: When high, it indicates wink of a right eye; when low, it indicates wink of a left eye; and when the center, it indicates no wink state.
- **Look Right/Left**: The sensitivity slider enables adjustment of the response sensitivity. When high, it indicates right sided tilt of eyes; when low, left-sided tilt of eye vision; and when the center, an indication of eyes looking straight ahead.
- **Raise Brow**: Low level means no raise brow detected. There is a rise in the signal level proportional to the strength of raise brow.
- **Furrow Brow**: Low level means no furrowed brow detected. There is a rise in the signal level proportional to the strength of furrow brow.
- **Smile**: Similar to raise brow and furrow brow, the low signal indicates no smile or neutral expression. The signal strength increases as smile is detected, proportional to the strength of the smile.
- **Clench**: The signal level is high whenever a clench is detected. Otherwise, it is low.
- **Right Smirk/Left Smirk**: With respect to a common graph line, the signal is low if there is a left smirk and the signal is high if there is a right smirk. A neutral position gives a centered signal output.
- **Laugh**: The output graph keeps on rising as a laugh is detected, according to its intensity.

3.6.2.3   Affectiv Suite

With the help of this suite, a user's real-time idiosyncratic emotions can be well analyzed and monitored. The three discrete recognition made by the Suite are engagement, instantaneous excitement, and long-term excitement. The Affectiv detections do not need any specific training for each user. It looks for universal brainwave characteristics. However, the user's data are used for calibration purpose in the existing program. The panel in Affectiv Suite contains two graphs for display of different combinations of detections and time scales. Timescale and color can be customized as per the need.

- **Instantaneous Excitement**

   This indicates the positive arousal of the user. The arousal can be physiological in nature. Common features throughout such a state are increasing the heart rate and muscle tensions, sweat gland stimulation, dilation of pupils, digestive, and blood flow inhibition. Almost all of these changes are related to the sympathetic nervous system.

- **Long-term Excitement**

   This is similar to instantaneous excitement but is for wider time periods. The time is usually considered in minutes.

- **Engagement**

This means the user is directing himself or herself toward responding a stimulus which demands some task. The user shows alertness and a conscious attitude. It is characterized by increased beta waves along with attenuated alpha waves and physiological arousal. The related emotions include alertness, vigilance, concentration, stimulation, and interest. The various API components of the EMOTIV EPOC headset are mentioned in Table 3.4.

3.7   Prior Work

In this section, a review has been provided on recent works related to brain–computer interface. In Birbaumer et al. (2000), a thought translation device (TTD) was developed for completely paralyzed patients using an operant learning approach for self-regulation of EEG signals using slow cortical potentials (SCPs) and the system was tried on five patients. Nakayama et al. (2007) give a brain–computer interface-based FFT and multilayer network and presents an analysis of features of brain waves extracted by the multilayer network. Five kinds of mental tasks have been analyzed, including baseline, multiplication, letter-composing, rotation of a 3D object and counting numbers. Same tasks have been again analyzed in Darvishi and Al-Ani (2007), and classification of these mental tasks has been done followed by statistical analysis. Imaginary left- and right-hand movements also provide particular EEG signals which have been analyzed using an adaptive neuron-fuzzy inference system (ANFIS) as the classification algorithm, having advantages like providing a set of parameters and linguistic rules that can be useful in interpreting the relationship between extracted features. The same has been analyzed in Nakayama and Inagaki (2006). It is quite important to know about the various algorithms of signal processing used to interface the brain with a machine. These have been discussed in a well-patterned manner in Lotte et al. (2007), Reaz et al. (2006), and Bashashati et al. (2007). A hand movement Control real-time system has been shown in Ahmadi and Erfanian (2009) done by the use of two classifiers are designed. The first classifier imagines movements of the right hand whereas the second classifier imagines the left-hand movements. Hand grasping, holding, and opening are covered by the classifier 1 and the classifier 2 performs error correction and activation of classifier 1. Singla and Haseena (2013) present a BCI-based wheelchair control system relying on steady-state visual evoked potentials and support vector machines in classification algorithms. Synthetic speech and typing have been made possible by Kennedy et al. (2000) without physical movement by an invasive technology of implantation of a special electrode into the outer layers of human neocortex. In Kim et al. (2007), Youngmin Kim et al. have used eye movements (electrooculogram signals/EOG) to develop a robust discrimination method in controlling a mobile robot and thus, successfully discriminating various eye movements using classification algorithm. In Millan et al. (2004), moving a mobile robot by a mere process of thinking has been

Table 3.4 List of API components in EMOTIV EPOC headset (Emotiv 2010)

API components	Description
Affectiv	Interprets the emotional state of the user
SDK neuroheadset	The user wears the neuroheadset on the scalp. The neuroheadset acquires electrical signals from the brain, amplifies them, and sends them to the EMOTIV EmoEngine
Cognitiv	This suite is primarily used when the user is in the state of consciousness
Default profile	Any new user is designated this profile with default settings which can be changed as per requirement
Detection	Expressiv, Affectiv, and Cognitiv suites can recognize definite states of the user including facial expressions, mental expressions, emotions, and thoughts. It is implemented by several high-level algorithms within the system called EMOTIV EmoEngine and the neuroheadset
EML (EmoComposer Markup Language)	This is a syntax based on XML. Its recognition can be done by the EmoComposer to command predefined mental states or EmoState values
EMOTIV application programming interface (API)	The API includes a vast function library which can be used by EMOTIV-based application developers while working with the EMOTIV neuroheadset and EMOTIV-based detection suites
EMOTIV EPOC	This name has been given to the headset which should be worn by the user for brain signal recognition
EMOTIV Software Development Kit (SDK)	The SDK enables application developers to develop games and applications by interacting with EMOTIVEmoEngine™ and EMOTIV neuroheadsets
EMOTIVSDKLite	It is a version of the EMOTIV SDK which allows integrating other software with the neuroheadset simulation
EmoComposer	This helps application developers speed up the process of EMOTIV EmoEngine emulation-based application development
EMOTIVEmoEngine	The EnoEngine helps managing settings specific to each user and each application while communication with the neuroheadset

(continued)

Table 3.4 (continued)

API components	Description
EmoKey	This is a simple tool that enables the user to relate their commands with traditional input devices such as the keyboard or the mouse
EmoScript	The EmoComposer can interpret this text file and relate the user's intentions to predefined EmoState
EmoState	This is kind of a dataset or a feature vector corresponding to a specific mental state or EMOTIV detection
Expressiv	The Expressiv Suite helps to identify the user's facial expressions and to classify them into the predefined ones
Profile	Each user who happens to use the neuroheadset is supposed to create their own profile which contains their data which in turn helps the EMOTIV control panel to perform better and detect better
User	The subjects who are wearing the neuroheadsets and use them to interact through their brain signals are called users. These people must have their own respective profiles

made possible by taking into consideration both user's thought and robot's perpetual state. At C4 and C5 levels of spinal cord injury, the system developed in Moon et al. (2005) can be taken into consideration which presents an electric-powered wheelchair driven by EMG (Electromyogram) signals generated by voluntary muscular contraction. Another wheelchair controlled by EEG signals has been presented in Tanaka et al. (2005) after developing a recursive training algorithm to generate recognition patterns from EEG signals.

The work in Cheemalapati et al. (2013) presents a real-time emotion detection algorithm using portable EEG and uses the Borealis stream processing engine in its implementation. A different technique of brain wave measurement is used in Girouard et al. (2013), namely, functional near-infrared spectroscopy (fNIRS) which measures the reemission of near-infrared light sent to the brain. The device deduces the behavior of brain activity from the bloodstream in the brain. It is a real-time system which effectively classifies workload states of the brain. An SSVEP-based BCI mind game has been proposed in Lalor et al. (2005), in which there is a common framework comprised of graphics, signal processing, and network communications. It also focuses on its importance on the rehabilitation of neurological disorders such as attention deficit/hyperactivity disorder. The classification algorithm used in Dobrea and Dobrea (2009) includes genetic algorithm-based ideology resulting in a better classification result and a faster BCI system. Khorshidtalab and Salami (2011) is an abstract review of the various classifications and feature extraction methods used in real-time EEG signal processing. The second part of our work focuses on the development of a mouse emulator to provide the user, the ability to move the pointer. A similar effort has been made in Rosas-Cholula et al. (2013) using EMOTIV software showing a gyroscope-driven mouse control. However, in Rosas-Cholula et al. (2013), Kalman filtering has been applied to the mouse position data of gyroscope. In our work, Kalman filtering has been done before the integration step (conversion from velocity into displacement).

References

Ahmadi, M., and A. Erfanian. 2009 April. An on-line BCI system for hand movement control using real-time recurrent probabilistic neural network. In *4th International IEEE/EMBS Conference on Neural Engineering, 2009, NER'09*, 367–370). New York: IEEE.

Aimone, C.A., A.S. Garten, S.E. Grant, O. Mayrand, T. Zimmermann, and Interaxon Inc. 2014. Brain sensing headband. U.S. Patent D709,673.

Aliki, M., and V. Emmanouel. 2008. *Polysomnography: Recent Data on Procedure and Analysis.* http://www.pneumon.org/assets/files/Archive/PNEUMON_2008-4.pdf#page=44.

Bashashati, A., M. Fatourechi, R.K. Ward, and G.E. Birch. 2007. A survey of signal processing algorithms in brain–computer interfaces based on electrical brain signals. *Journal of Neural Engineering* 4 (2): R32.

Birbaumer, N., A. Kubler, N. Ghanayim, T. Hinterberger, J. Perelmouter, J. Kaiser, I. Iversen, B. Kotchoubey, N. Neumann, and H. Flor. 2000. The thought translation device (TTD) for completely paralyzed patients. *IEEE Transactions on Rehabilitation Engineering* 8 (2): 190–193.

Cheemalapati, S., M. Gubanov, M. Del Vale, and A. Pyayt. 2013, August. A real-time classification algorithm for emotion detection using portable EEG. In *2013 IEEE 14th International Conference on Information Reuse and Integration (IRI)*, 720–723. New York: IEEE.

Cincotti, F., D. Mattia, C. Babiloni, F. Carducci, S. Salinari, L. Bianchi, M.G. Marciani, and F. Babiloni. 2003. The use of EEG modifications due to motor imagery for brain-computer interfaces. *IEEE Transactions on Neural Systems and Rehabilitation Engineering* 11 (2): 131–133.

Darvishi, S., and A. Al-Ani. 2007, August. Brain-computer interface analysis using continuous wavelet transform and adaptive neuro-fuzzy classifier. In *Engineering in Medicine and Biology Society, 2007. EMBS 2007. 29th Annual International Conference of the IEEE*, 3220–3223. New York: IEEE.

Dobrea, D.M., and M.C. Dobrea. 2009, November. Optimisation of a BCI system using the GA tehnique. In *2nd International Symposium on Applied Sciences in Biomedical and Communication Technologies, 2009. ISABEL 2009*, 1–6. New York: IEEE.

Emotiv, S.D.K. 2010. *Research Edition Specifications.*

Girouard, A., E.T. Solovey, and R.J. Jacob. 2013. Designing a passive brain computer interface using real time classification of functional near-infrared spectroscopy. *International Journal of Autonomous and Adaptive Communications Systems* 6 (1): 26–44.

Graimann, B., B. Allison, and G. Pfurtscheller. 2009. Brain–computer interfaces: a gentle introduction. In *Brain-Computer Interfaces*, 1–27. Berlin: Springer.

Kennedy, P.R., R.A. Bakay, M.M. Moore, K. Adams, and J. Goldwaithe. 2000. Direct control of a computer from the human central nervous system. *IEEE Transactions on Rehabilitation Engineering* 8 (2): 198–202.

Khorshidtalab, A., and M.J.E. Salami. 2011, May. EEG signal classification for real-time brain-computer interface applications: a review. In *2011 4th International Conference on Mechatronics (ICOM)*, 1–7. New York: IEEE.

Kim, Y., N.L. Doh, Y. Youm, and W.K. Chung. 2007. Robust discrimination method of the electrooculogram signals for human-computer interaction controlling mobile robot. *Intelligent Automation & Soft Computing* 13 (3): 319–336.

Lalor, E.C., S.P. Kelly, C. Finucane, R. Burke, R. Smith, R.B. Reilly, and G. Mcdarby. 2005. Steady-state VEP-based brain-computer interface control in an immersive 3D gaming environment. *EURASIP Journal on Applied Signal Processing* 2005: 3156–3164.

Lotte, F., M. Congedo, A. Lécuyer, F. Lamarche, and B. Arnaldi. 2007. A review of classification algorithms for EEG-based brain–computer interfaces. *Journal of Neural Engineering* 4 (2): R1.

Mahajan, R., D. Bansal, and S. Singh. 2014. A real time set up for retrieval of emotional states from human neural responses. *International Journal of Medical, Health, Pharmaceutical and Biomedical Engineering* 8 (3): 142–147.

Mason, S.G., and G.E. Birch. 2000. A brain-controlled switch for asynchronous control applications. *IEEE Transactions on Biomedical Engineering* 47 (10): 1297–1307.

Millan, J.R., F. Renkens, J. Mourino, and W. Gerstner. 2004. Noninvasive brain-actuated control of a mobile robot by human EEG. *IEEE Transactions on Biomedical Engineering* 51 (6): 1026–1033.

Moon, I., M. Lee, J. Chu, and Mun, M. 2005, April. Wearable EMG-based HCI for electric-powered wheelchair users with motor disabilities. In *Proceedings of the 2005 IEEE International Conference on Robotics and Automation, 2005. ICRA 2005*, 2649–2654. New York: IEEE.

Nakayama, K., and K. Inagaki. 2006, December. A brain computer interface based on neural network with efficient pre-processing. In *International Symposium on Intelligent Signal Processing and Communications, 2006. ISPACS'06*, 673–676. New York: IEEE.

Nakayama, K., Y. Kaneda, and A. Hirano. 2007, November. A brain computer interface based on FFT and multilayer neural network-feature extraction and generalization. In *International Symposium on Intelligent Signal Processing and Communication Systems, 2007. ISPACS 2007*, 826–829. New York: IEEE.

Ramoser, H., J. Muller-Gerking, and G. Pfurtscheller. 2000. Optimal spatial filtering of single trial EEG during imagined hand movement. *IEEE Transactions on Rehabilitation Engineering* 8 (4): 441–446.

Reaz, M.B., M.S. Hussain, and F. Mohd-Yasin. 2006. Techniques of EMG signal analysis: detection, processing, classification, and applications. *Biological Procedures Online* 8 (1): 11–35.

Rosas-Cholula, G., J.M. Ramirez-Cortes, V. Alarcon-Aquino, P. Gomez-Gil, J.D.J. Rangel-Magdaleno, and C. Reyes-Garcia. 2013. Gyroscope-driven mouse pointer with an EMOTIV® EEG headset and data analysis based on empirical mode decomposition. *Sensors* 13 (8): 10561–10583.

Signal, N.B. 2015. NeuroSky, Inc. http://neurosky.com/Year.

Singla, R., and B.A. Haseena. 2013. BCI based wheelchair control using steady state visual evoked potentials and support Vector machines. *International Journal of Soft Computing and Engineering (IJSCE)* 3 (3): 46–52.

Tanaka, K., K. Matsunaga, and H.O. Wang. 2005. Electroencephalogram-based control of an electric wheelchair. *IEEE Transactions on Robotics* 21 (4): 762–766.

Ungureanu, M., C. Bigan, R. Strungaru, and V. Lazarescu. 2004. Independent component analysis applied in biomedical signal processing. *Measurement Science Review* 4 (2): 18.

Wolpaw, J.R., N. Birbaumer, D.J. McFarland, G. Pfurtscheller, and T.M. Vaughan. 2002. Brain—computer interfaces for communication and control. *Clinical Neurophysiology* 113 (6): 767–791.

Wolpaw, J.R., G.E. Loeb, B.Z. Allison, E. Donchin, O.F. do Nascimento, W.J. Heetderks, F. Nijboer, W.G. Shain, and J.N. Turner. 2006. BCI meeting 2005-workshop on signals and recording methods. *IEEE Transactions on Neural Systems and Rehabilitation Engineering* 14 (2): 138–141.

Chapter 4
Implementation

Abstract The proposed system comprises of three main parts, the first one being the wireless acquisition module, second is the signal processing module and the third, the last one is the output hardware module in which the user inputs get implemented as the final desired outputs. The following Fig. 4.1 shows the overall block diagram of the system implemented in our work. The workflow can be mainly classified into two parts. The first part is the electroencephalogram (EEG) acquisition and signal processing in real time. As shown in Fig. 4.1 next, the left side of the block diagram covers the first part of our work that is data acquisition, signal processing, and implementation of this processed data into real-time robot commands. The data that is referred to include only the raw EEG data provided by various electrodes in the EMOTIV EPOC neuroheadset. The second part of our work is acquisition, processing, and implementation of the gyroscope signals. Here, the gyroscope that is referred to is embedded in the EMOTIV EPOC neuroheadset. This has been mentioned on the right-hand side of the block diagram which can also be named as the mouse emulator part, that is, the data from the gyroscope is used to drive the mouse pointer on the computer to access the GUI in MATLAB. The third part is the design of GUI in MATLAB, shown in the right, bottom corner of the block diagram, which is to be concentrated upon by the user. When the abovementioned sections work at the same time simultaneously, the user can access his GUI in MATLAB to communicate with the Arduino-based autonomous navigation robot in real time.

4.1 Specifications Used

EMOTIV Research Edition Premium 1.0.0.5 application programming interface (API) has been used in the implementation as it allows the extraction of raw EEG data from the neuroheadset.

The EMOTIV software development kit (SDK) is comprised of one or two SDK neuroheadsets, installation CD and one or two USB wireless receivers. The users' brainwaves are captured by the neuroheadset and converted into digital form. Afterward, the brainwaves are sent to the USB receiver after some preprocessing. EMO-

© The Author(s), under exclusive license to Springer Nature Singapore Pte Ltd. 2019   57
S. Das et al., *Real-Time BCI System Design to Control Arduino Based Speed Controllable Robot Using EEG*, SpringerBriefs in Computational Intelligence,
https://doi.org/10.1007/978-981-13-3098-8_4

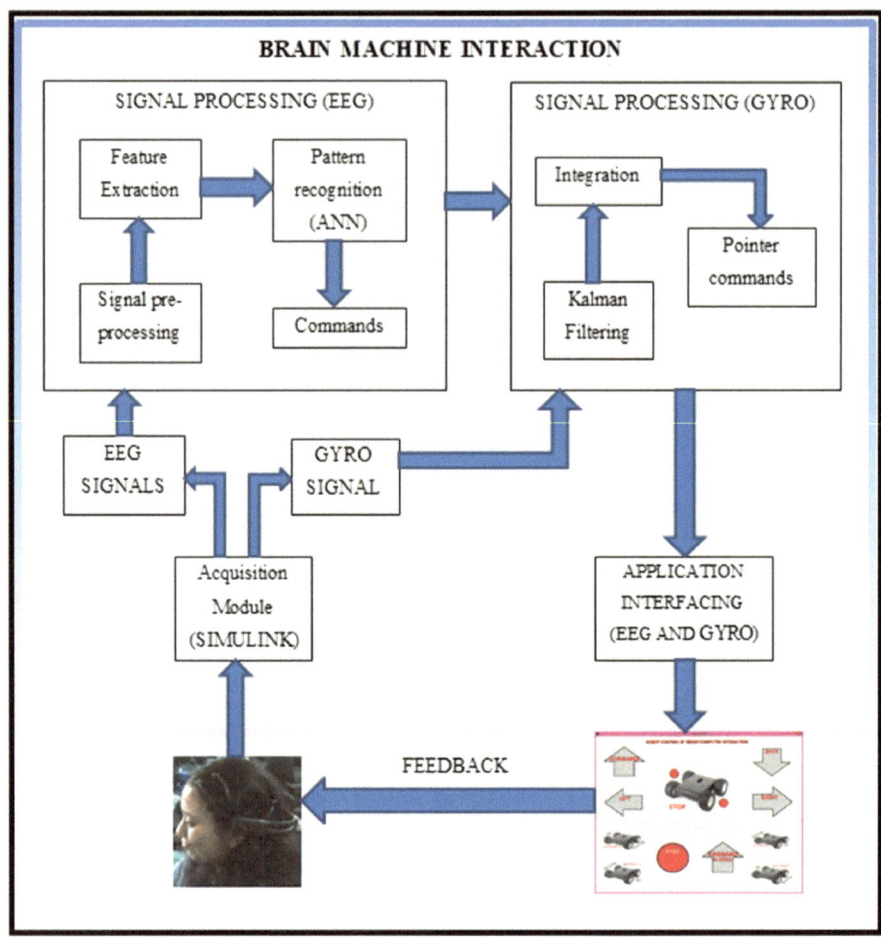

Fig. 4.1 Flow diagram of the system designed as the per working process (figure generated by the authors)

TIVEmoEngine is a post-processing software which needs to be installed in the PC to apply the results obtained from the acquisition system to the EMOTIV application programming interface (API). The PC specifications are as follows:

- Intel Xeon processor (3.4 GHz, 16 GB RAM)
- 64-bit Windows 8.1 operating system
- MATLAB 2013b.

4.2   Acquisition

4.2.1   Signal Quality Check

The process of acquisition starts with the user putting on the neuroheadset correctly. The headset is switched on and then the Bluetooth dongle is connected to the PC for wireless reception of EEG information from the user's scalp to the computer. When the Control Panel is viewed on the PC, the user first must select the corresponding user ID (needs to be created in case of new users). This displays the contact qualities of the electrodes, in the EMOTIV Control Panel, thereby providing guidance on how to get the best quality signal from the electrode contact. It is vital for the user to maintain quality contact for a better quality of classification of EEG. The following Fig. 4.2 depicts various contact qualities achieved in the neuroheadset during a session. Each circle represents a single sensor on the user's scalp along with the approximate location of the sensor. The quality of each contact is denoted by the color of its representative circle. Various colors along with their significance are given below (Table 4.1):

It must be tried that every electrode gives a status of green in the Control Panel. Only after the verification of signal quality, the user can proceed to the next step.

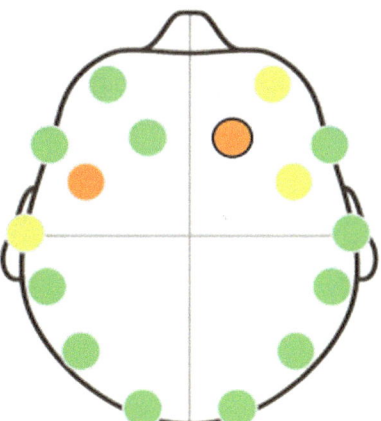

Fig. 4.2 Signal quality of EMOTIV EPOC (figure generated by the authors during experimental sessions, Emotiv 2010)

Table 4.1 Signal quality color representation (Emotiv 2010)

Representing color	Signal quality
Black	No signal
Red	Very poor signal
Orange	Poor signal
Yellow	Fair signal
Green	Good signal

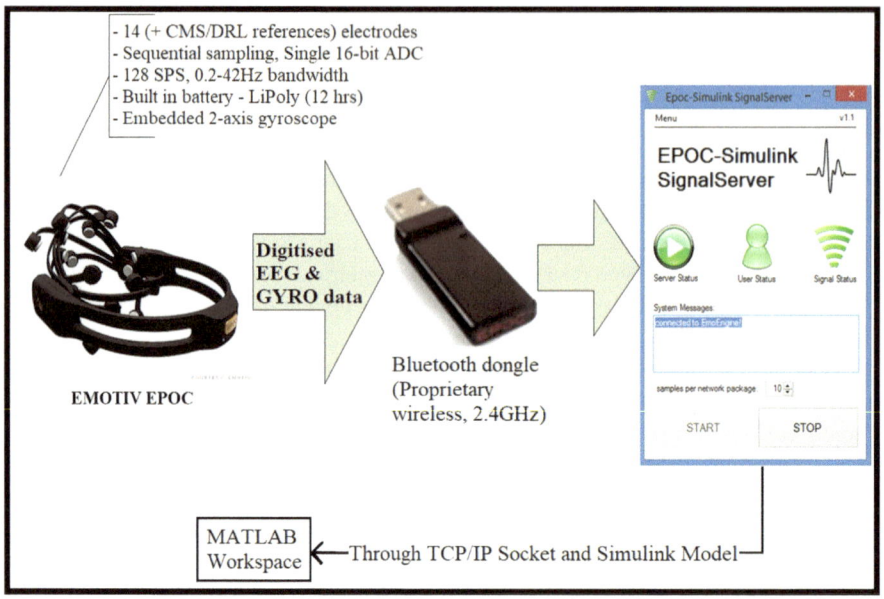

Fig. 4.3 Process of acquisition in detail (figure generated by the authors)

As shown in Fig. 4.3, the EMOTIV EPOC headset contains a single 16-bit ADC for conversion of the raw EEG and GYRO signals that are obtained in the analog domain into digital format. It uses a sampling frequency of 128 Hz. The headset also contains a 2-axis gyroscope embedded inside for detecting displacement of the headset in two axes, *x* and *y*. The built-in battery is of LiPoly type that can last for 12 h in working condition. Thus, a digitized form of EEG and GYRO data is acquired from the neuroheadset which is transmitted to the computer through a Bluetooth dongle. The wireless communication between the neuroheadset and the Bluetooth dongle takes place through some unknown proprietary method (in the name of EMOTIV). Next, the EPOC SIMULINK server helps to acquire all information into MATLAB SIMULINK. The EPOC server sends data to SIMULINK S-Function using a TCP/IP socket.

4.2.2 SIMULINK EEG Importer Interfacing for Online Acquisition of Data

The EPOC SIMULINK EEG Importer has been used in order to acquire real-time EEG data from the EMOTIV EPOC headset to a MATLAB SIMULINK model. After successful installation of the EPOC SIMULINK Importer, the files, edk.dll, and edk_utils.dll are copied from *C:\Program Files (x86)\EMOTIV Research Edi-*

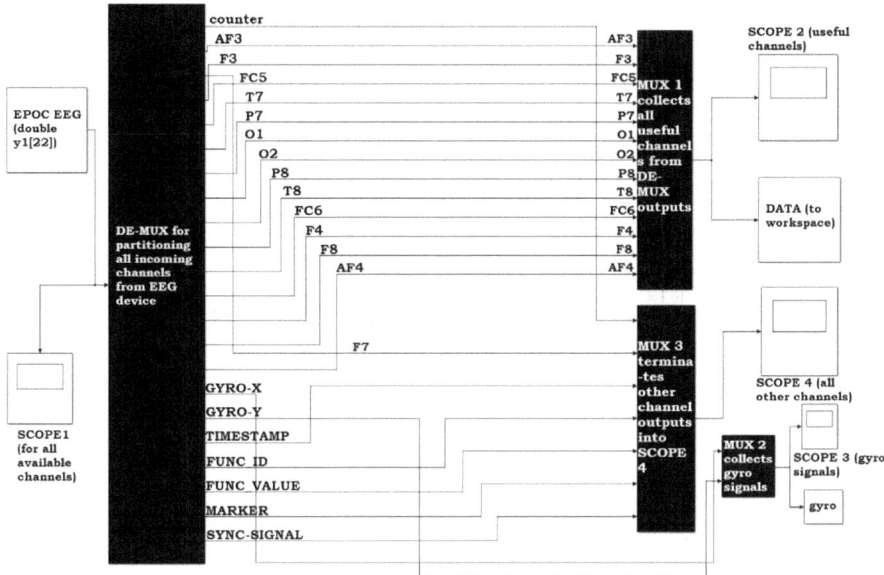

Fig. 4.4 Signal acquisition model through SIMULINK (figure generated in SIMULINK by the authors)

tion SDK v1.0.0.5-PREMIUM to *C:\Program Files (x86)\EpocSIMULINK EEG Importer*.

Next, after achieving green signals in all electrodes as in the Control Panel, the EpocSignalServer (Fig. 4.5) from the desktop is started and the START button in the EpocSignalServer window is pressed. This shows green colored icons in the server status, user status, and signal status.

MATLAB is started next and the current working folder/directory is changed to the EPOC SIMULINK EEG Importer installation folder, that is, *C:\Program Files (x86) \EpocSIMULINK EEG Importer/MATLAB*. Next, the SIMULINK model, that is, compatible with the MATLAB version in use is started and the model is edited as per need. The model is named *EMOTIVEpocEEG_testmodel_2012b.mdl*. However, a few simulation settings are necessary before proceeding as listed down:

- Change the solver options type from variable step to fixed step.
- Set the solver at discrete (no continuous states) state.
- Set the fixed-step size (fundamental sample time) at 1/128 as the sampling frequency of EPOC headset is 128 Hz.

Figure 4.4 shows the complete SIMULINK model for extraction of EEG data from the Importer to MATLAB workspace. First of all, a SIMULINK block receives the EEG data in vector format, that is, the EPOC EEG block on the left-hand side. The incoming signals can be observed in the SCOPE1 which depicts all the available channels. Figure 4.5 shows the EPOC SIMULINK Server Control Panel which the

Fig. 4.5 EPOC SIMULINK
Server Control Panel
showing signal status (figure
captured by the authors
during experimental
sessions, Emotiv 2010)

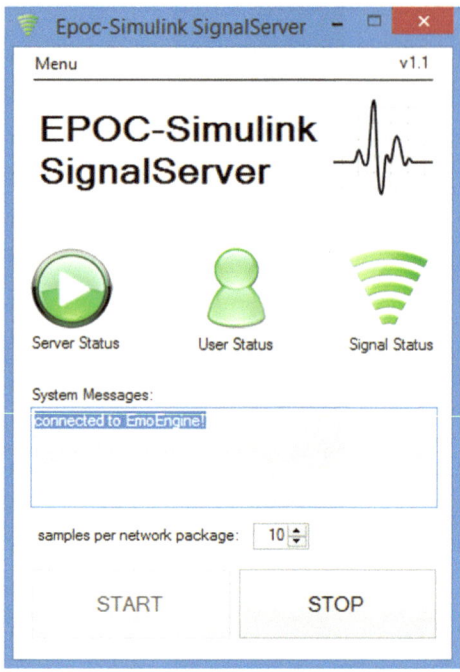

Fig. 4.5 EPOC SIMULINK
Server Control Panel
showing signal status (figure
captured by the authors
during experimental
sessions, Emotiv 2010)

enables the real-time acquisition and monitoring of the EEG and gyro signals. The
de-mux (demultiplexer) extracts the components of the input signals and outputs
these components as separate signals as shown in Fig. 4.6. On the other hand, the
mux (multiplexer) combines its inputs into a single vector output, which is easier to
work upon in MATLAB. Thus, the overall function of the de-mux and mux is that
they extract the useful channels from the input vector and output these channels as a
single vector.

The acquired data can be further processed in the SIMULINK environment.
SIMULINK block, thus used is created out of a MATLAB MEX S-function and
outputs a double data vector of size (McFarland and Wolpaw 2008). This vector is in
the format of: COUNTER, AF3, F7, F3, FC5, T7, P7, O1, O2, P8, T8, FC6, F4, F8,
AF4, GYRO-X, GYRO-Y, TIMESTAMP, FUNC ID, FUNC VALUE, MARKER,
and SYNC SIGNAL. Figure 4.7 shows the output waveforms from SCOPE 1 before
demultiplexing. Next, the acquired vector is partitioned as unique individual signals
by the use of a demultiplexer as shown in Fig. 4.6. Afterward, the useful channels
can be extracted from this vector. Using two multiplexers, the useful channels are
separated from rest that is, using MUX 1 and MUX 3. MUX 2 is to extract the
GYRO-X and GYRO-Y signals separately into a workspace variable. SCOPE 2 can
be used to view all the useful channels in real time, which are: AF3, F3, FC5, T7,
P7, O1, O2, P8, T8, FC6, F4, F8, and AF4 (Fig. 4.8).

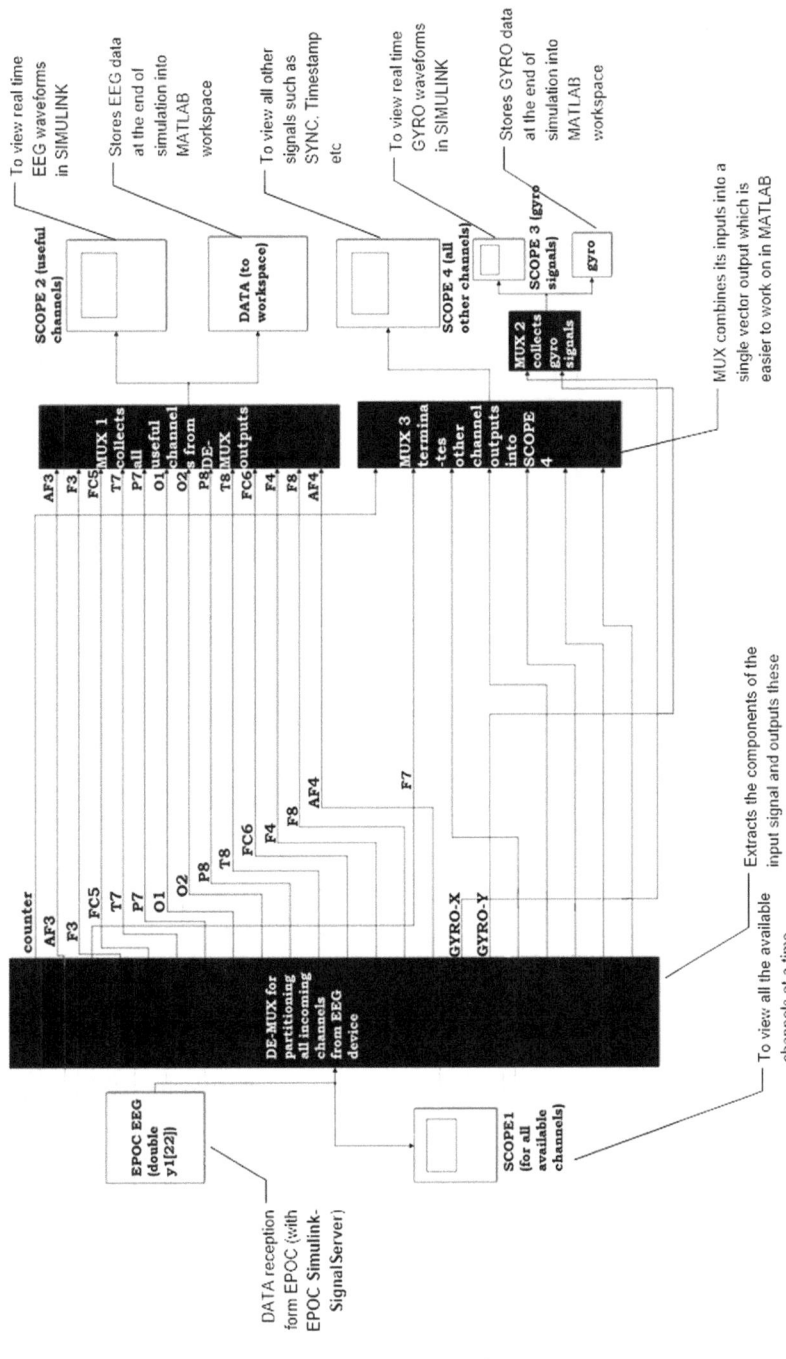

Fig. 4.6 Detailed SIMULINK model in operation (figure generated in SIMULINK by the authors)

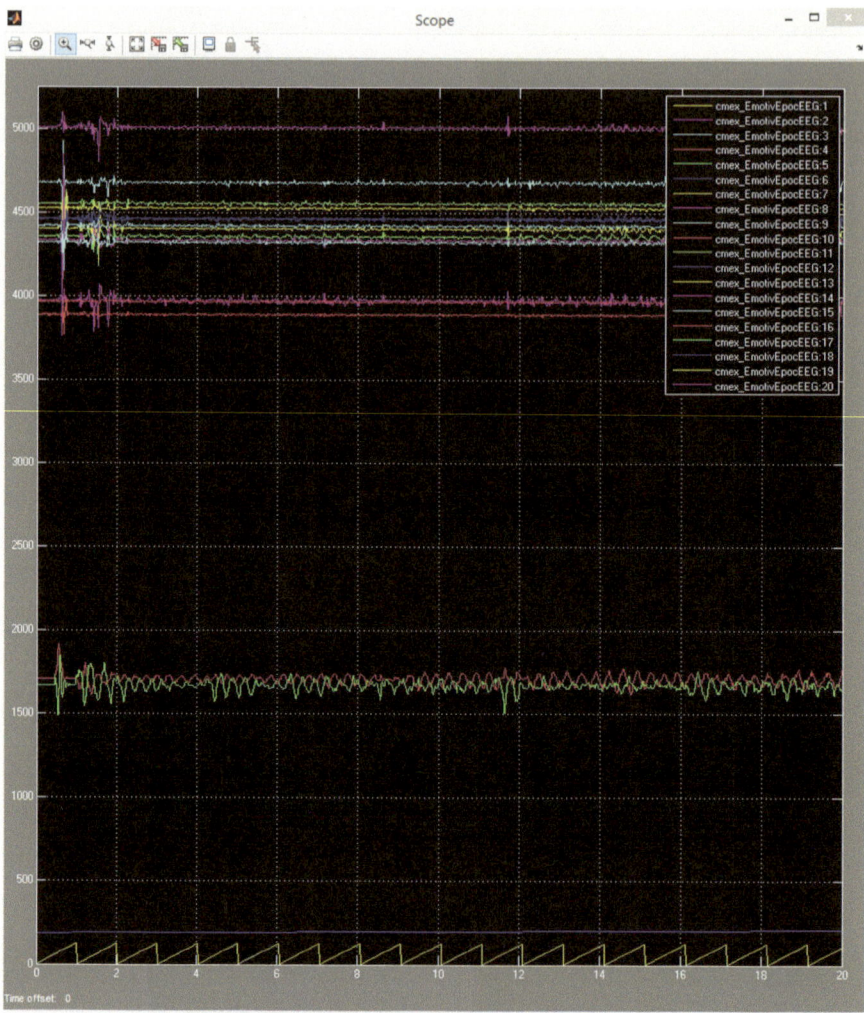

Fig. 4.7 SCOPE 1 waveforms (all available channels along with gyro signals and packet data status signal; figure captured during experimental sessions)

The channel F7 is ignored in our system as it got disrupted due to some mishandling by the users. Similarly, SCOPE 4 can be used to view the rest of the channels that include COUNTER, TIMESTAMP, FUNC ID, FUNC VALUE, MARKER, and SYNC SIGNAL.

SCOPE 3 can be used to view the gyroscope signals which show the movement of the user's head in X-and Y-axis simultaneously (Fig. 4.9).

Signals that are to be used further for signal processing are stored in a Workspace variable in the MATLAB workspace as shown in Fig. 4.6. The SIMULINK block

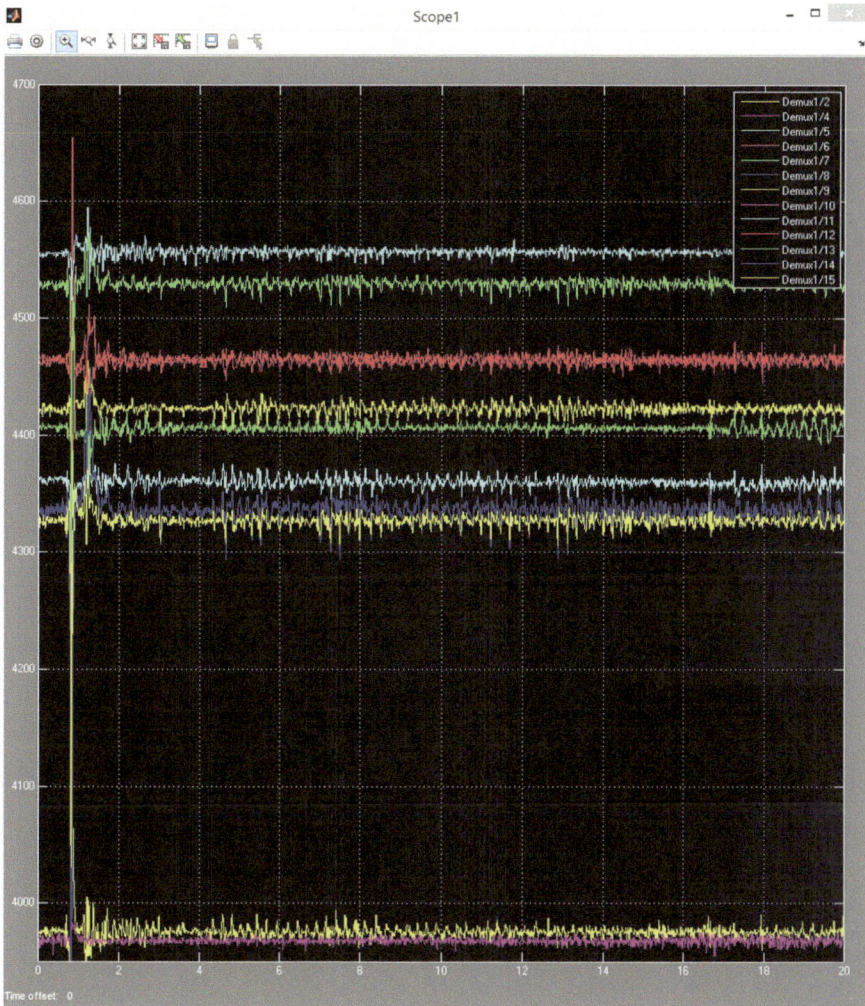

Fig. 4.8 SCOPE 2 waveforms showing 13 useful channels extracted by a demultiplexer (figure captured during experimental sessions)

used for the same is the "To Workspace" block. For use of the model in real time, it is run for 0.5 s and then terminated. On termination, the model stops running and the workspace variables get updated. These data can be used for further steps of processing and then, the model is run for another 0.5 s for the next set of data, and so on.

For offline acquisition of data used for training purpose, the EMOTIV Testbench software can also be used. It allows the collection of data over a given period of time

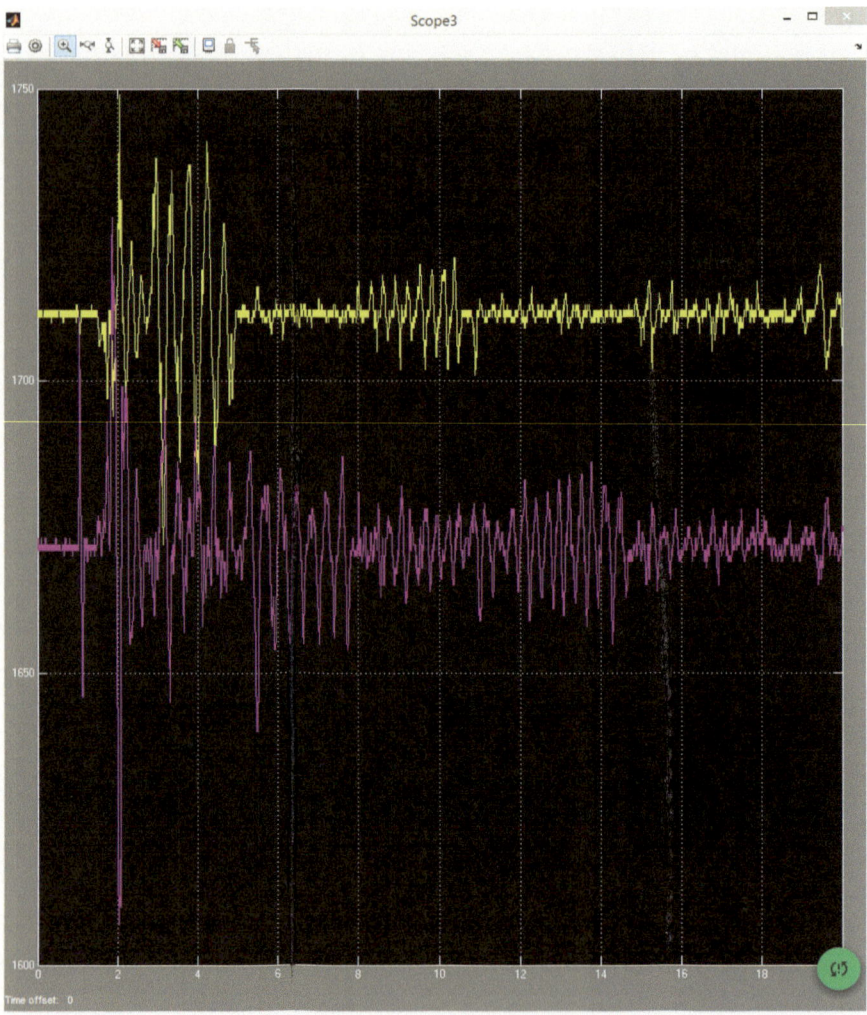

Fig. 4.9 SCOPE 3 showing the gyroscope movement sensing signals in X and Y axes (figure captured during experimental sessions)

into.edf (European data format) form. This data can be converted into .csv (Comma separable value) form which can be easily read in MATLAB for further processing.

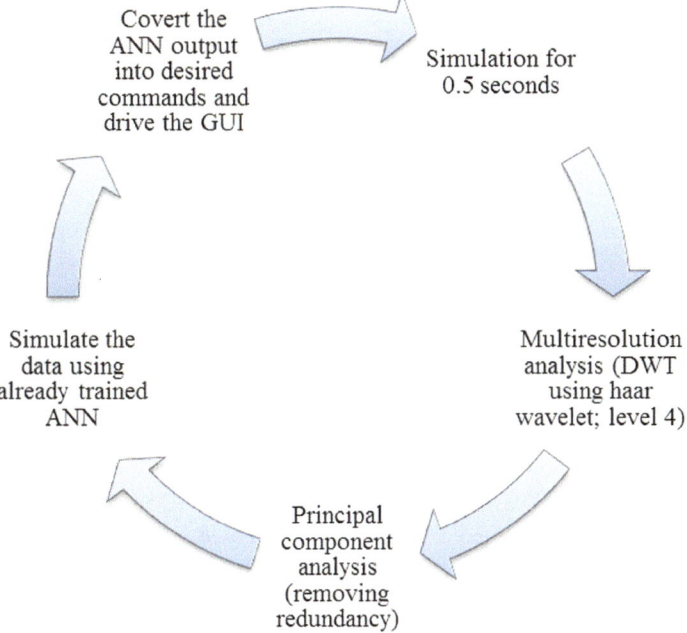

Fig. 4.10 Flow diagram of EEG signal classification module in detail (figure generated by the authors)

4.3 EEG Data Classification Module

The cycle shown in Fig. 4.10 is followed by the classification algorithm for classifying EEG data. Firstly, simulation in SIMULINK helps acquisition of data from the neuroheadset for 0.5 s. This data is processed by level 4 multi-resolution analysis resulting in DWT coefficients in the next stage. Out of these coefficients, the optimal one is chosen for principal component analysis (PCA), in order to remove redundancy from the signal. Then it is simulated by the neural network for the purpose of classification into the type of data it belongs to. Once the classification is done, the system comes to know about the intention of the user through his/her EEG and hence accordingly, drives the GUI in MATLAB for commanding the autonomous Arduino-based robot.

All the processes mentioned in the block diagram above have been described below.

Table 4.2 List of Subjects

Subject	Age	Gender
Subject 1	23	Female
Subject 2	24	Male
Subject 3	27	Male

4.3.1 Signal Processing and Classification Algorithm

Preprocessing is done in order to lift up the quality of signals so that they can be made eligible to be processed in the subsequent steps. In our work, preprocessing has been done in the neuroheadset itself. No separate preprocessing has been done. The EMOTIV Testbench software displays the electroencephalographic data in real time along the fourteen monitored channels. Signals vary each time the user thinks something in a conscious or an unconscious manner. Variations may also be observed due to electromyographic data, such as facial expressions (smile, raise brow) and electrooculographic data, such as looking left, looking right, blinking, etc. The data obtained from Testbench software is used in order to form databases for four different classes namely, smile, raise a brow, neutral, and blink. This database is collected from three different subjects or users. Two of them are male and all of them are in the age range of 20–30 years (Table 4.2).

Ten trials for each class are made. The EMOTIV Testbench software gives the display of EEG data in real time, which can be stored by the user as per the required time period. Each trial is partitioned from the other by two minutes of rest. This is necessary as the user is to be brought to a stable condition before making him/her perform the next action.

The data obtained from the Testbench software is in .edf format and is converted into.csv format by the Testbench software itself. The .csv file thus obtained contains 36 columns of data in total. The first row contains a header notation. Columns 3–16 are the EEG readings of 14 channels. The other 22 columns of data are those gathered from preprocessed data. The rows denote the number of samples collected in the given time period. Since the sampling frequency used in EMOTIV EPOC is 128 Hz, 128 samples are obtained in 1 second. This means that a recording of 2 min gives us $128 * 2 * 60 = 15{,}360$ samples.

In the next step, the unwanted data are removed from the .csv file and the 14-channel data are extracted into a MATLAB variable. Three databases are created for extracted data for the subjects separately. An important point to be noted is that, for creating databases, the samples from the duration 0.5–1.5 min are to be considered only. This is done because, whenever data is collected, the first and last 0.5 min has the possibility of containing the maximum amount of noise and randomness.

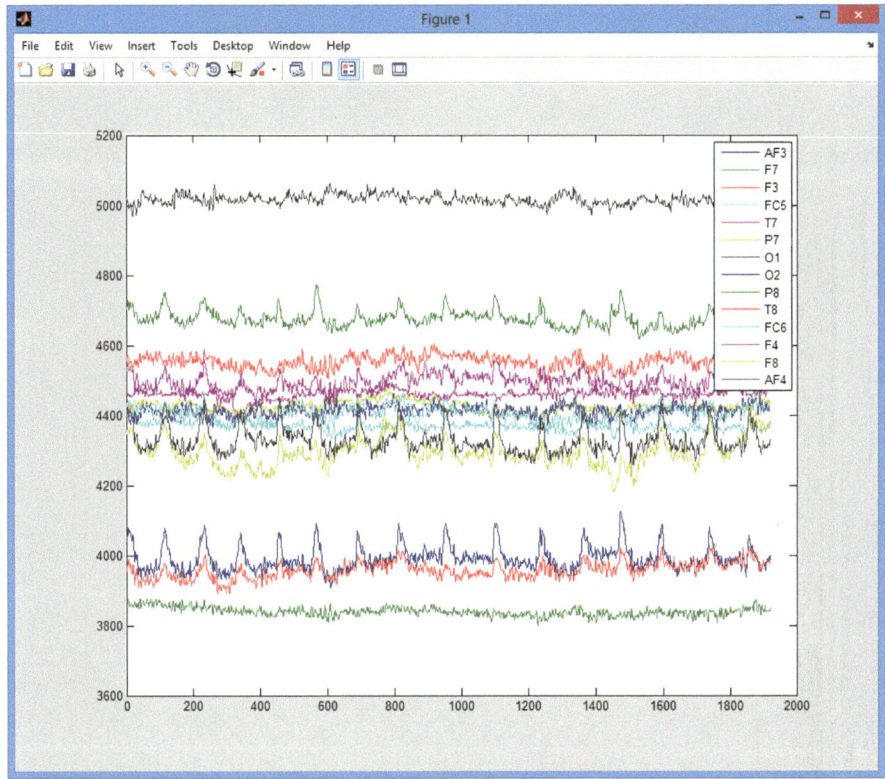

Fig. 4.11 Blink waveform of all 14 channels shown in MATLAB (figure captured during experimental sessions)

4.3.2 Analysis of Data

The behavior of the 14 channels can be observed by plotting them separately in MATLAB for each class. The following figures denote 0.25 min (1920 samples depicting 15 s) of data representing each of blink, raisebrow, smile, neutral data along with the channels where distinct variations can be found in each expression (Fig. 4.11 to Fig. 4.17).

Blink can be seen in the P300 wave in the above waveforms. The clear variations are mostly observed in AF3, F7, O1, F4, and AF4 channels (Fig. 4.12). It can be seen in the form of a sudden peak and then, a fall in the wave.

Raise Brow is also a P300 wave seen in the Fig. 4.13. A sudden rise in the wave is followed by a slow falling with another probable peak in the mid. Maximum variations are observed in AF3, F3, T7, O1, FC6, and F8 channels (Fig. 4.14).

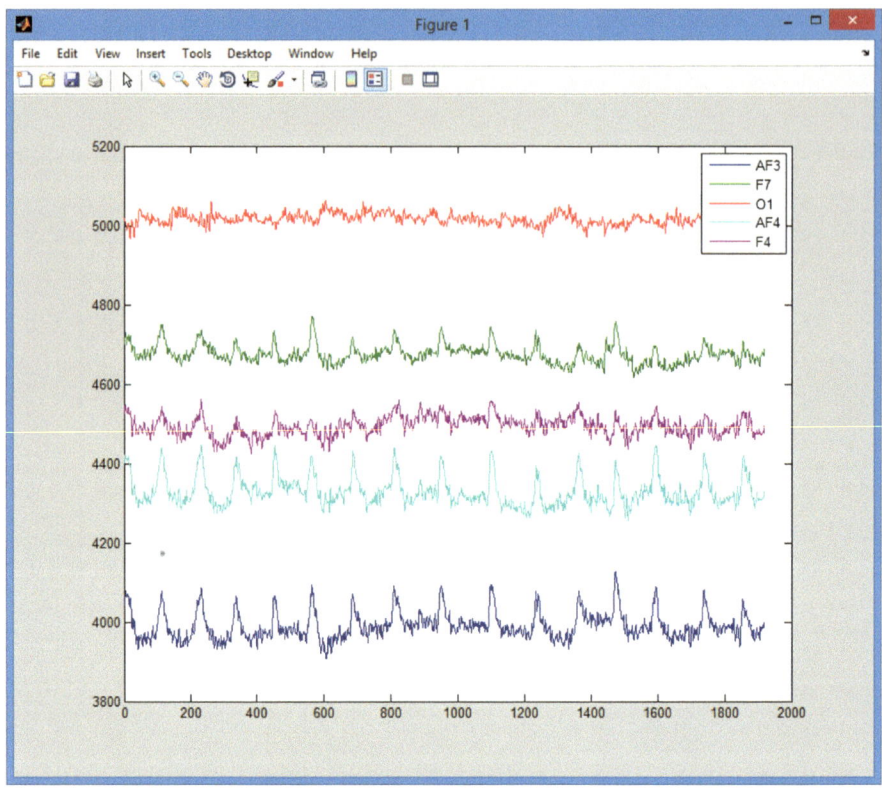

Fig. 4.12 Channels where blink is distinctly visible as compared to others (figure captured during experimental sessions)

Smile signal is more of a random signal with several peaks in single smile signal intent of the user. Most variations are observed in F3, AF3, T7, T8, AF4, and FC6 channels (Figs. 4.15 and 4.16).

The neutral signal (Fig. 4.17) is observed in the system by making the subjects stay calm without any facial expressions or movements. The signal thus obtained shows no variable changes in all the channels.

4.3.3 Observations

It has been observed from the above studies that the distinct changes can be viewed only in a few channels that include all except O2 and P8. Training of neural networks is tried with and without the inclusion of the data obtained from these channels. It was observed that better classification accuracies could be obtained after the inclusion of all the channels without ignoring any of them in particular. So, the final training

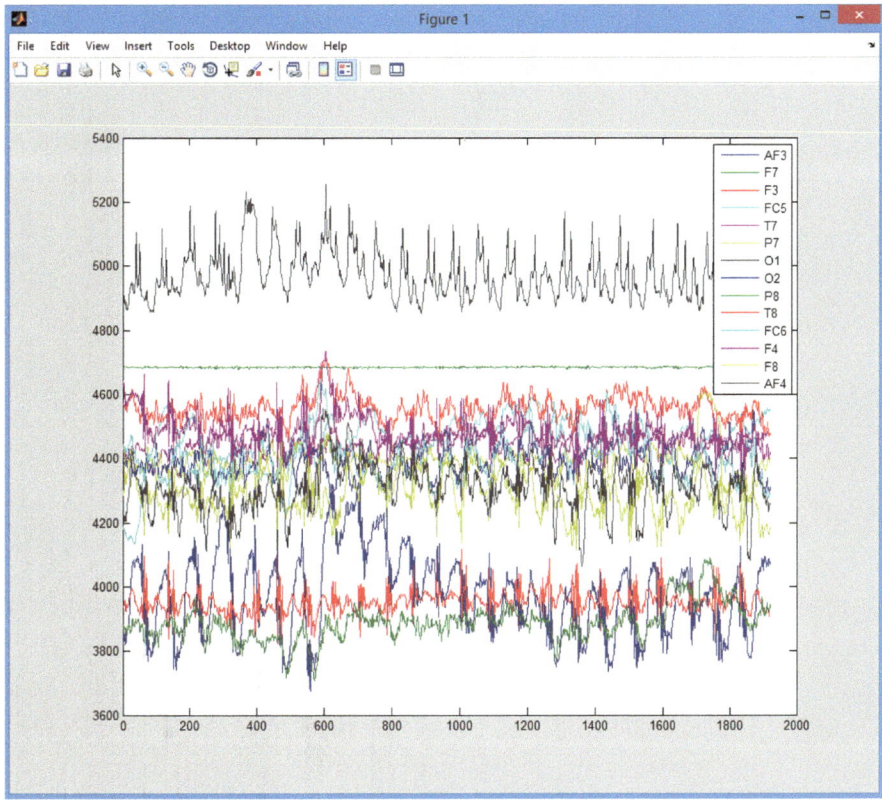

Fig. 4.13 Raise brow waveform of all 14 channels shown in MATLAB (figure captured during experimental sessions)

was done without neglecting the data from any of the channels. Otherwise, this step of reducing the number of channels could have been named as a feature extraction step.

4.3.4   DWT Analysis

The classification algorithm starts with a multi-resolution analysis of the samples to split the signal into different frequency ranges and examine their efficacy.

These signals can further be analyzed by applying Fourier transform and hence gathering the frequency components present in the signal. Short-time Fourier Transform gives us an idea of where in time the spectral components appear in the signal. The sampling frequency of our system is 128 Hz. Now, according to Nyquist criterion, the sampling rate, fs is twice the highest frequency component in the signal.

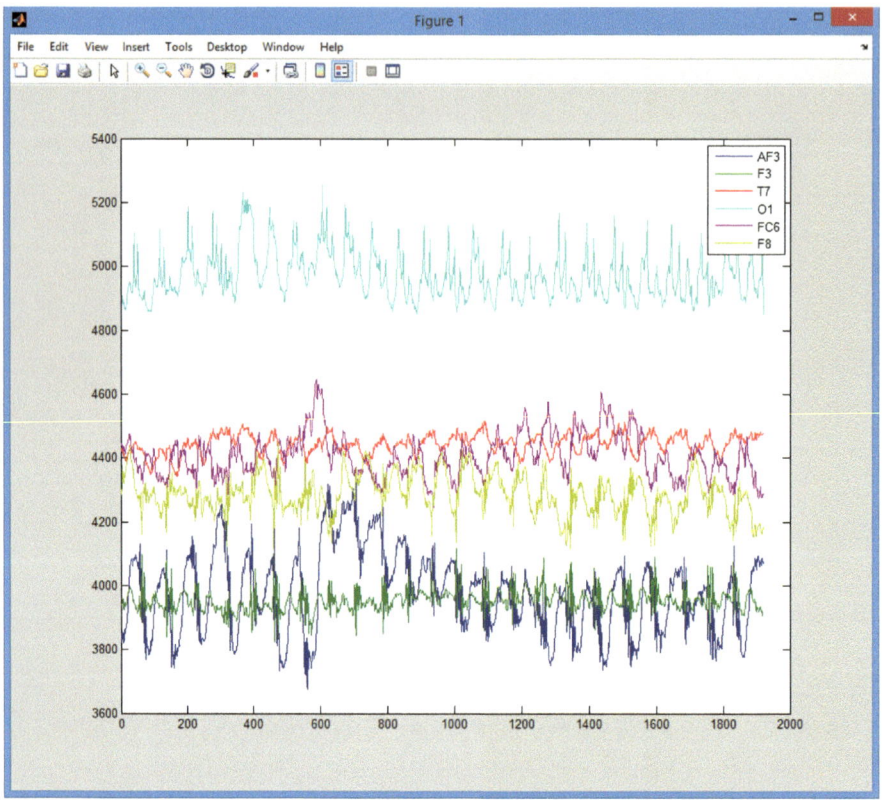

Fig. 4.14 Channels where raise brow is distinctly visible as compared to others (figure captured during experimental sessions)

This concept can be used to conclude that the highest frequency present in the signal essentially is 64 Hz (=128/2 Hz). This gives us an idea of applying multi-resolution analysis to split the signal in various frequency ranges and thus easy analysis of classification accuracy of various actions in those frequency bands. Figure 4.18 shows the whole process of multi-resolution analysis. It starts with our source signal $x[n]$ that contains frequency components of (0–64) Hz. This signal is split into five frequency ranges:

- (0–4) Hz
- (4–8) Hz
- (8–16) Hz
- (16–32) Hz
- (32–64) Hz.

Four levels of decomposition give these five ranges of frequencies.

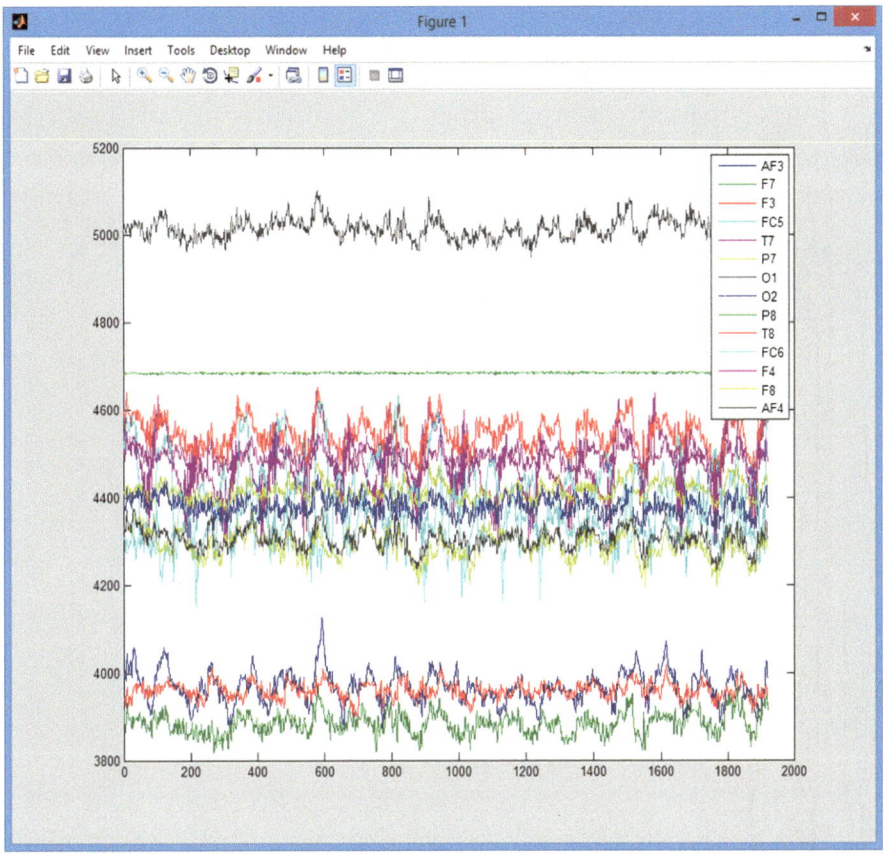

Fig. 4.15 Smile waveform of all 14 channels shown in MATLAB (figure captured during experimental sessions)

- In the first level, $x[n]$, the source signal is passed through a low-pass filter ($h[n]$) and a high-pass filter ($g[n]$). This results in two frequency components ranging (32–64) Hz—high-frequency component and (0–64) Hz—low-frequency component. Then after, downsampling by a factor of two is done, which results into two DWT coefficients.
- The coefficient obtained by passing the signal through a high-pass filter ($g[n]$) and downsampled by two is called the "Detailed coefficient (D)".
- The coefficient obtained by passing the signal through a low-pass filter ($h[n]$) and downsampled by two is called the "Approximation coefficient (A)".
- In the next level, level 2, a similar process is repeated with source signal being the approximation coefficient from level 1 in place of $x[n]$ as in level 1.
- Repetition of a similar process for four levels will provide four detailed coefficients, $D1$ (32–64) Hz, $D2$ (16–32) Hz, $D3$ (8–16) Hz, and $D4$ (4–8) Hz.
- An approximation coefficient is obtained from level 4, $A4$ (0–4) Hz.

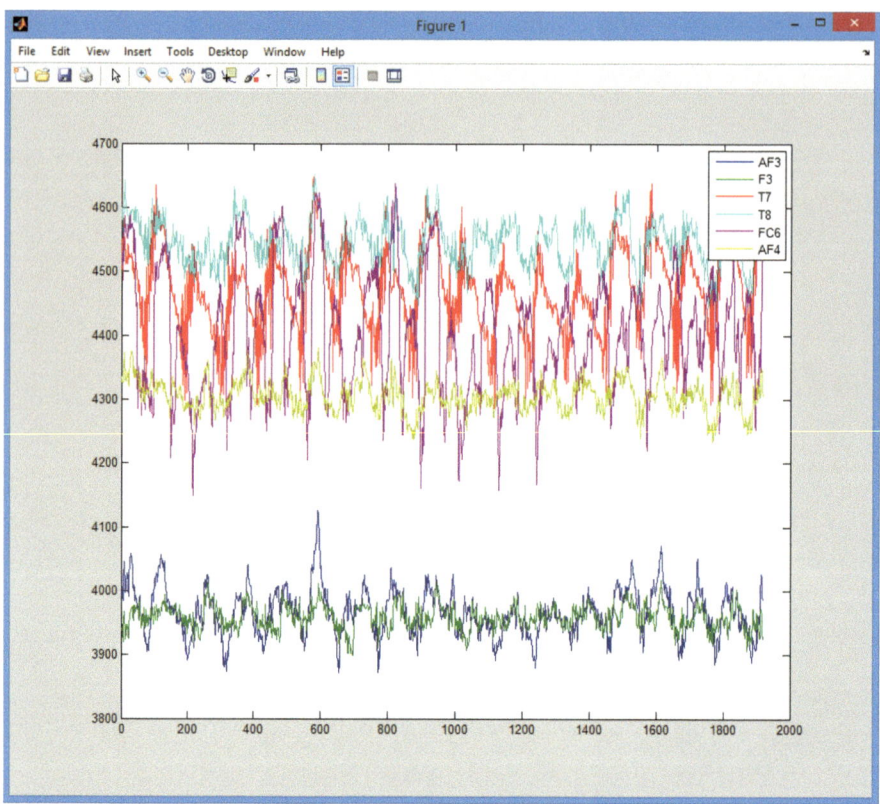

Fig. 4.16 Channels where smile is distinctly visible as compared to others (figure captured during experimental sessions)

The various ranges of frequencies in the EEG that can be linked to actions and different stages of consciousness are given here. An interesting point to be noted is that the DWT coefficients obtained by multi-resolution analysis share nearly the same ranges of frequencies as of the EEG frequency ranges, shown below:

- Gamma waves (31 Hz and up): This range reflects the mechanism of consciousness.
- Beta and Gamma waves show traits of attention, perception, and cognition.
- Beta waves (12–30 Hz): These are small and fast waves associated with focussed concentration and are dominant in the central and frontal areas of the brain.
- Alpha waves (7.5–12 Hz): Alpha waves are comparatively slower and are associated with relaxation and disengagement that are dominant in the frontal lobe and the back part of the brain.
- Theta waves (3.5–7.5 Hz): Theta waves are associated with inefficiency, daydreaming, frustration, emotional stress or disappointment, deep meditation, and creative inspiration. The lower levels of theta waves represent the line between awake and

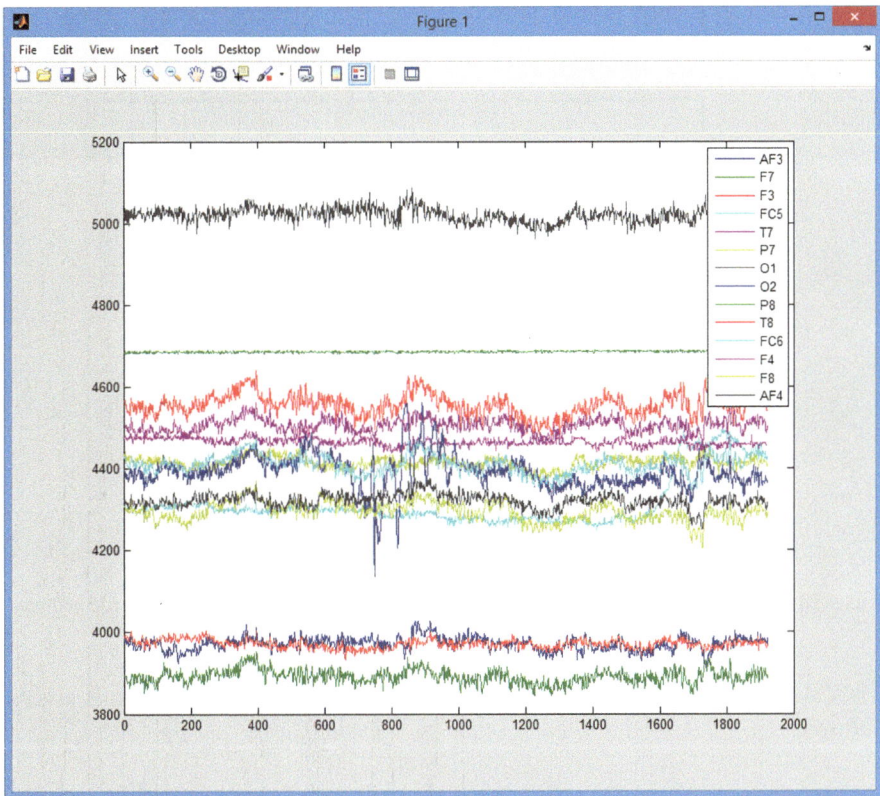

Fig. 4.17 Neutral waveform of all 14 channels shown in MATLAB (figure captured during experimental sessions)

sleep state. However, higher levels of theta waves represent abnormalities in adults generally related to attention deficit/hyperactivity disorder (AD/HD).

- Delta waves (0.5–3.5 Hz): These are generally the slowest waves that occur when sleeping. If these waves occur when a person is awake, physical defects are assumed in the brain.

After level 4 DWT analysis in the algorithm, five frequency range signals are obtained as mentioned earlier, of which four are detailed coefficients and one approximation coefficient. The beta ($D2$) range of waves is chosen after multi-resolution. This is because beta waves are associated with focussed concentration related to the frontal and central areas of the brain. When a patient operates the GUI, these waves are witnessed to be the most dominant. The wavelet family used in our algorithm is "haar" which has been chosen after a prolonged study of obtained accuracies. Haar wavelet comprises of certain sequences of rescaled "square-shaped" functions forming a wavelet family altogether. It was proposed for the first time by Alfred Haar in

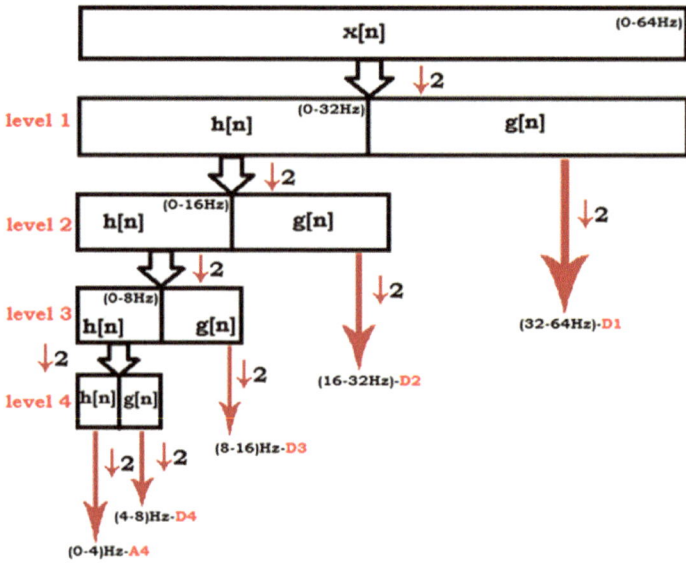

Fig. 4.18 Multi-resolution analysis in pictorial representation (figure generated by the authors)

1909 (Haar 1911). The mother wavelet $\psi(t)$ of Haar wavelet transform is given as follows:

$$\psi(x) = \begin{cases} 1 & 0 \le x \le \frac{1}{2} \\ -1 & \frac{1}{2} < x \le 1 \\ 0 & \text{otherwise} \end{cases} \quad \text{(Haar 1911)} \tag{4.1}$$

$$\psi_{jk}(x) \equiv \psi\left(2^j x - k\right) \quad \text{(Haar 1911)} \tag{4.2}$$

The obtained signal after applying DWT is then processed with principal component analysis (PCA) in order to remove correlations between the data.

4.3.5 PCA

The principal component analysis (PCA) is a method that can sometimes be used as a signal enhancer or can be applied for dimensionality reduction post feature extraction (Wold et al. 1987). PCA can also effectively find patterns in data which contain multiple variables for consideration, some of them probably being irrelevant. It is primarily a dimensionality reduction technique. It is one of the best methods for spotting the uniqueness or variability of the data. It converts the high dimensional data into lower dimensions by the method of projection of the least squares, capturing major inconsistencies, and ignoring minor inconsistencies. Before using PCA, it is important to standardize the input data by making the resultant mean, null.

PCA is a simple, nonparametric method that helps the extraction of germane datasets from raw information. The main intention of this procedure is to highlight the similarities and differences of the input data in order to spotlight the important patterns (Wold et al. 1987).

$$\text{Variation explained by each Principal Component} = \frac{\text{Sum of Eigen Value}}{\text{Number of Variables}} \text{ (Wold et al. 1987)}$$

$$(4.3)$$

4.3.6 Neural Networks

Neural networks are based on self-learning algorithms which do not require programming skills of a programmer. The neural network models imitate the mechanism of biological processing of information in the human neural system. These models comprise of a set of inputs and outputs which are nonlinearly mapped with each other. The mapping is adaptive in nature.

Artificial neural networks (ANNs) are comprised of electronic processing elements (PEs) connected in a peculiar pattern. Its behavior is dependent upon the weights of the trained ANN. ANNs are quite advantageous over conventional electronic processing techniques which include flexible learning techniques, the ability of generalization, distributed memory, parallel processing, and redundancy.

In this work, the neural network has been used for pattern recognition. Pattern recognition, now, is one of the most successfully emerged applications of ANN. As shown in the following Fig. 4.19, the neural network under use has been developed with the help of MATLAB toolbox, comprising of 10 hidden neurons, classifying 2 types of output data. The input data contains vectors of size 13. In other words, each sample contains 13 sets of data in it.

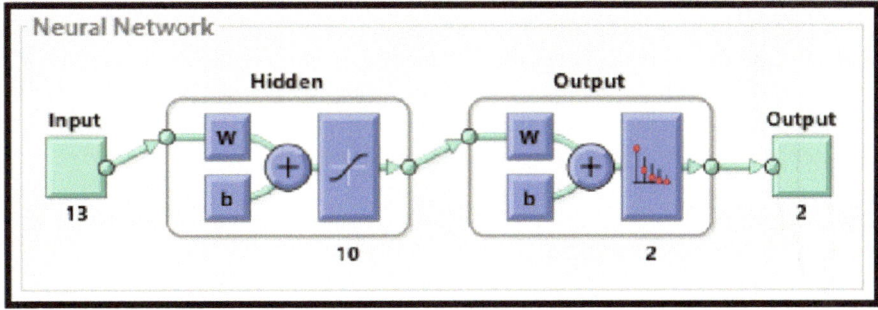

Fig. 4.19 Neural network format designed in MATLAB (figure captured during experimental sessions)

Scaled conjugate gradient has been used in this algorithm. Various ranges of frequencies have been tested upon for better classification accuracies as shown below. The figures shown later in this section depict confusion matrices of ANN training in alpha, beta, gamma, delta and theta ranges of frequencies in two subjects, 1 and 2. Training: Cross-Validation: Testing Ratio is set at 90:5:5.

4.3.6.1 Scaled Conjugate Gradient Algorithm

Scaled conjugate gradient algorithm is a subdivision of the conjugate gradient methods of feedforward neural network classification algorithms. The class of conjugate gradient methods (CGMs) comprises of second-order techniques which minimize multiple variable goal functions. The technical meaning of second order functions is that the second order derivatives of the goal function are used by these methods; while on the other hand, the first-order techniques make use of the first-order derivatives. Standard backpropagation techniques can be classified as first-order techniques. Out of the two variants, the performance of second-order techniques is better than first-order techniques when it comes to finding a way to the local minimum. Even after using second order information, SCG requires only $O(N)$ memory usage, where N is the number of weights in the neural network. However, a great disadvantage is its higher computational cost. It needs to compute the response of the network to each set of training input, several times before confirming the network's final makeover (Scaled Conjugate Gradient 2017). SCG algorithm is specifically designed for avoiding consumption of ample time for line searching. This algorithm is a combination of the model-trust region approach and the conjugate gradient approach together. There is no line search performed during each iteration. Speeding up of this algorithm depends upon the convergence criterion. The more accuracy needed, the higher speed is followed. SCG is a fully automated algorithm requiring no user-dependent parameters.

CGMs, just like other standard backpropagation methods, use an iterative process to reach the minimum value. The direction of iteration of conjugate gradient method is the conjugate of the directions of previous steps. This property makes it different from standard backpropagation methods. In the case of standard backpropagation methods, the direction is always along the error function gradient. In addition to it, each step of iteration is independent of the other in case of CGMs. For standard backpropagation methods, there are instances when the minimization achieved in one step of iteration is undone by the next step, although partially, and so on.

4.3.6.2 Main Features of SCG

The scaled conjugate gradient method of neural network classification differs from other conjugate gradient algorithms in two main aspects as given below.

In each iteration k, weight w_k is computed such that the new conjugate direction is R^N and the step size in this direction is $w_{k+1} = w_k + \alpha_k \cdot p_k$. p_k is eventually dependent on α_k. Here, α_k is the Hessian matrix of the error function. In other conjugate gradient methods, the evaluation of α_k is simply done by a tedious procedure. SCG, on the other hand, computes the Hessian matrix by simple approximation of the error term $E^{\prod}(w_k)$.

SCG also uses a scalar α_k that can control the vagueness of the Hessian matrix so that there is no possibility of the Hessian not being a positive definite, preventing the algorithm from achieving good performance.

SCG has contributed to both the fields of optimization theory and neural learning and is also considered faster than standard backpropagation and other conjugate gradient methods.

4.3.6.3 Parameters of SCG

Computation of parameters $s_k = \frac{E'(w_k + \sigma_k \cdot p_k) - E'(w_k)}{\sigma_k} + \lambda_k \cdot p_k$ and λ_k are dependent on their respective values at step $k - 1$. There are two main initial parameters of SCG namely, the initial values λ_k and σ_k. These values are dependent on the respective conditions λ_k and σ_1. Based on observations, Moller has proved that bigger values of $0 < \sigma_1 \leq 10^{-4}$ can cause a time taking convergence. The third parameter λ_1 varies from $0 < \lambda_1 \leq 10^{-6}$ (can be compared to standard backpropagation).

Termination of the learning process of a neural network is usually determined by the user. Unfortunately, the σ_1 mechanism sometimes leads to assigning of too large values to Δ_{max} in cases when further progress is difficult. To overcome floating-point exceptions, a termination criterion is added to SCG based on a few CGMs. SCG has an important advantage of being a batch learning method which makes it immune to pattern shuffling.

The confusion matrix generated in MATLAB contains significant information on its own. Four matrices are generated at a time. They all are for different sets of data. The first matrix is for the training set, next is for the validation data set. Next, two are for test data set and an overall confusion matrix, respectively (Fig. 4.20).

The above diagram is an example of a generic confusion matrix. It can be explained in detail as follows. There are three classes of data in total. Hence, three rows and three columns can be observed for the given data. The first column depicts the class 1 targets. There were seven class 1 targets in total out of which, six were assigned correctly to the output class 1 depicted as green in color. The rest 1 data is assigned incorrectly to the output class 2 due to which it is shown in red color. 0 entries were classified to the output class 3, which can thus be ignored. Now, the percentage accuracy of classification for class 1 data can be calculated as $6/7 * 100 = 85.7\%$ shown in GREEN in the first column bottom box. Incorrect assignment of data is similarly represented in RED that can be calculated as $1/7 * 100 = 14.3\%$. Similar readings can be taken from the other output classes for their corresponding columns. The overall accuracy is calculated as the percentage of input data that are correctly classified out of the total number of input data. In this case, 22 data are correctly classified out of 27 data which gives an overall accuracy of $22/27 * 100 = 81.5\%$.

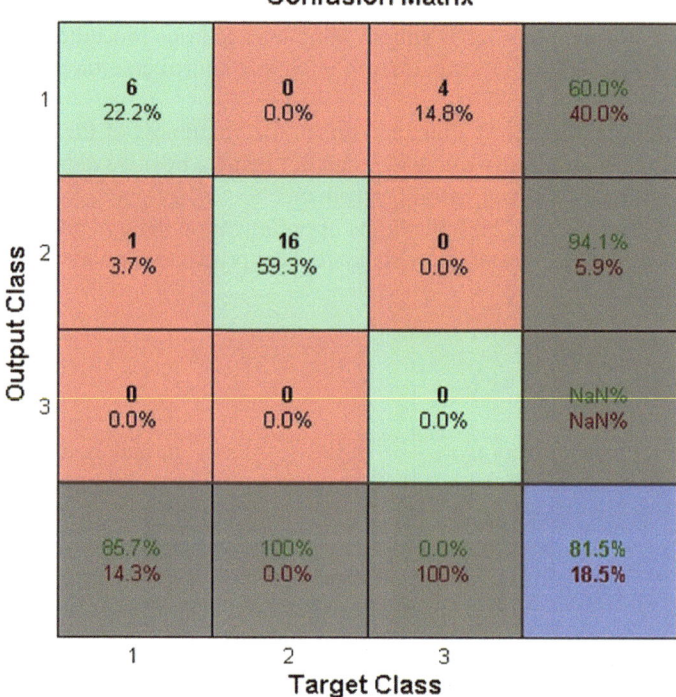

Fig. 4.20 Confusion matrix example (figure captured during experimental sessions)

This value has been shown in the box of the confusion matrix. The diagonal elements shown in GREEN depict the correctly classified data in all the three classes.

Subject 1 training confusion matrices and performance graphs (Figs. 4.21, 4.22, 4.23, 4.24 and 4.25):

Subject 2 training confusion matrices and performance graphs (Figs. 4.26, 4.27, 4.28, 4.29 and 4.30):

It has been clearly observed from the above confusion matrices that maximum classification accuracies are obtained in the beta and gamma ranges of frequencies. The theoretical explanation behind this is that beta waves are linked with focused concentration and the gamma waves are linked with traits of consciousness which are both dominant when the user is interacting with the GUI in MATLAB.

A higher accuracy has been obtained in the case of subject 1.

The database obtained during the acquisition phase of implementation is used in sections in order to train the neural network as shown till now. An important point to be noted is that the valuable samples from the database are first subdivided into sections of 64 samples before applying the necessary steps of signal processing. After the application of signal processing steps to those 64 sample sets of data, those

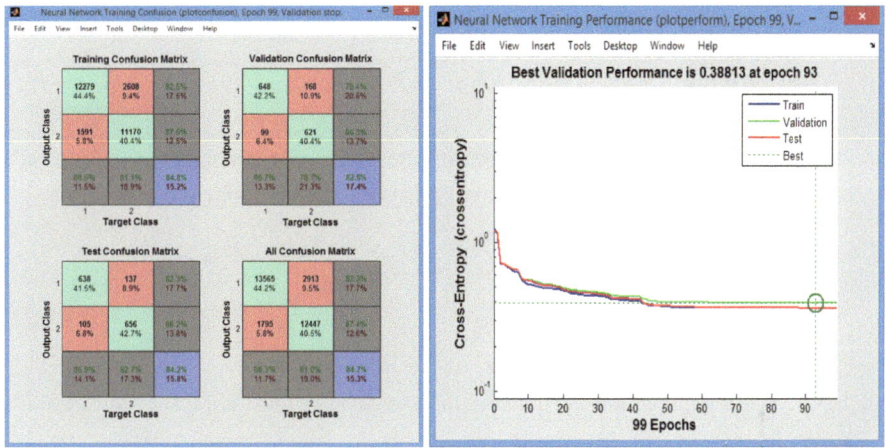

Fig. 4.21 Confusion matrix and performance plot in Subject 1 alpha frequency range (figure captured during experimental sessions)

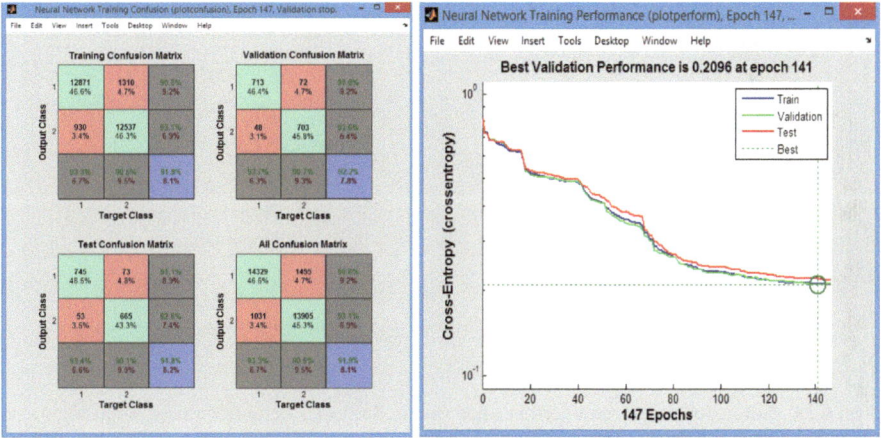

Fig. 4.22 Confusion matrix and performance plot in Subject 1 beta frequency range (figure captured during experimental sessions)

applied to the training session of the neural network. We obtain the accuracies of classification as mentioned in this section.

Now, the best trained neural network is fed with the same size of 64 processed data samples in the real-time domain via SIMULINK. On doing the same, we receive a classified output at the same time and can process it further as a decision maker in the MATLAB GUIs designed to control robots as shown in the next section.

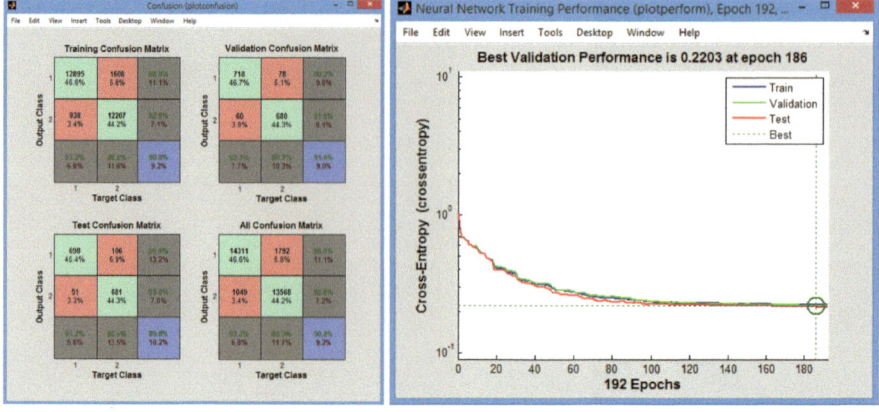

Fig. 4.23 Confusion matrix and performance plot in Subject 1 gamma frequency range (figure captured during experimental sessions)

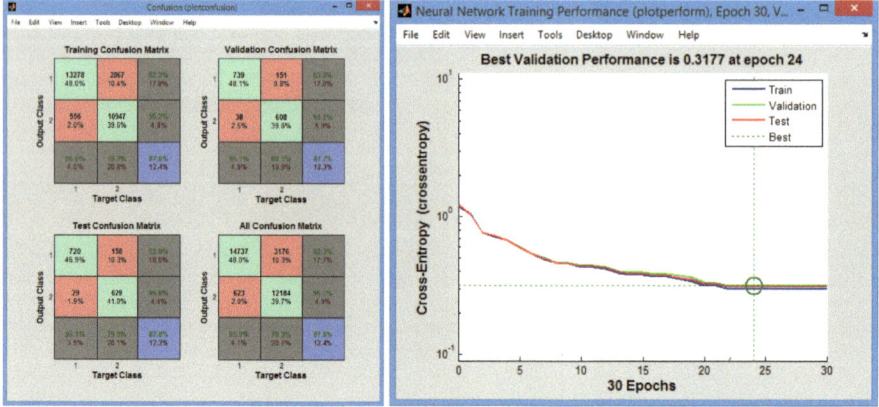

Fig. 4.24 Confusion matrix and performance plot in Subject 1 delta frequency range (figure captured during experimental sessions)

4.4 Gyroscope Signal Processing

It was observed that the gyroscope embedded in EMOTIV EPOC neuroheadset is designed to provide the angular velocity (rate of change of the angular position over time) measured in deg/s. The velocity data was then passed through a Kalman filter to remove unwanted noise and jitter. The Kalman filter operates as a state estimator for input data and helps taking care of jitter or high-frequency noise. Figure 4.31 shows the repetitive method followed in order to implement the mouse emulator.

Kalman is a recursive predictive filter that is based on the principle of covariance error reduction, thereby behaving as an ideal estimator. It is also termed as a Bayesian filter as it is based on recursive Bayesian estimation. The filter basically estimates

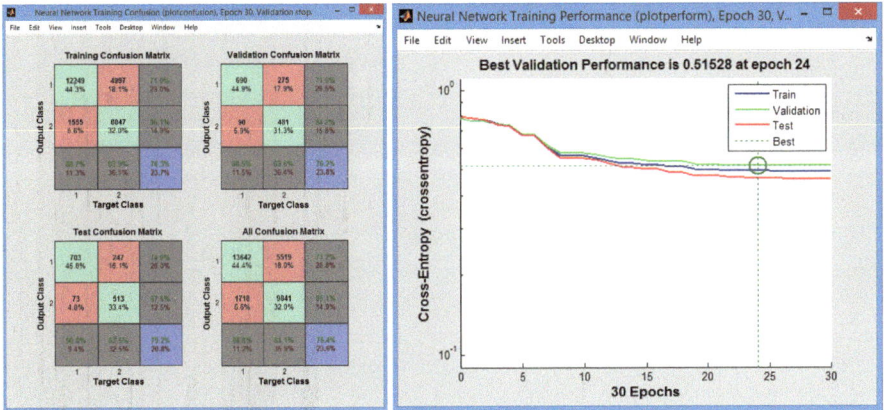

Fig. 4.25 Confusion matrix and performance plot in Subject 1 theta frequency range (figure captured during experimental sessions)

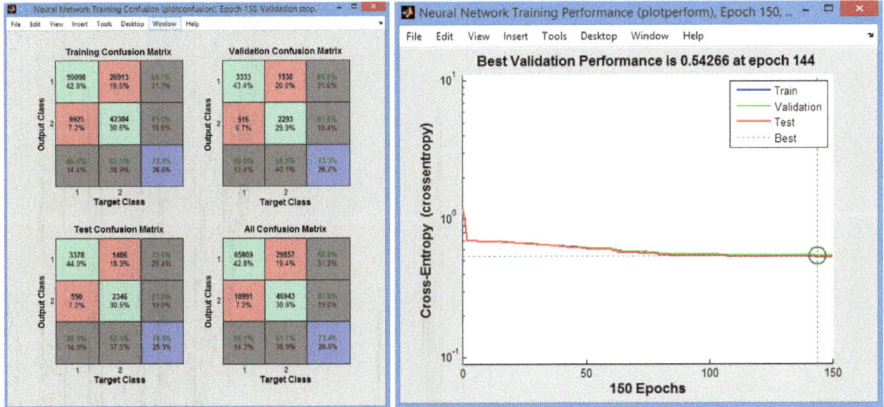

Fig. 4.26 Confusion matrix and performance plot in Subject 2 alpha frequency range (figure captured during experimental sessions)

the future states of an active system based on noisy incoming signals, considered as measurements, from the gyroscope. A continuous repetition of this process leads to a lessening of the estimated covariance error between the estimated state and the measurement. A new estimate of system's present state is calculated using the previous time step's state estimate and the present time step's measurement. Consider an object moving in a straight path but affected by random uncontrollable forces. If its position is measured every T_s second, but the measurements being affected by those uncontrollable forces, a model can be developed to depict the movement of that object.

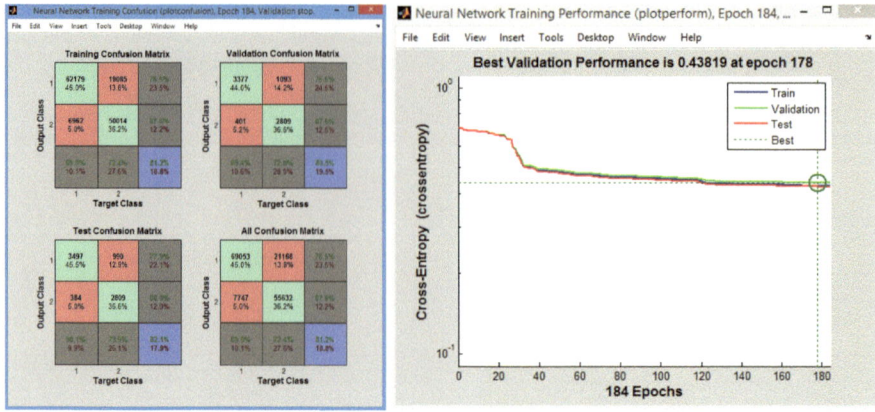

Fig. 4.27 Confusion matrix and performance plot in Subject 2 beta frequency range (figure captured during experimental sessions)

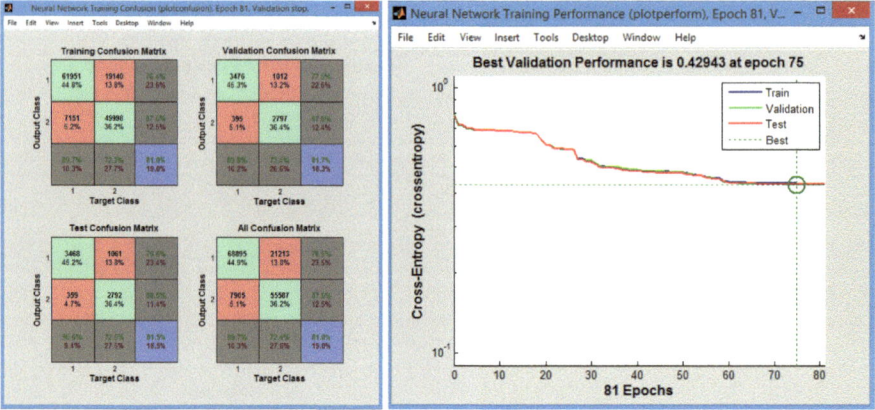

Fig. 4.28 Confusion matrix and performance plot in Subject 2 gamma frequency range (figure captured during experimental sessions)

$$\text{State transition matrix, } A = \begin{bmatrix} 1 & 0 & T_s & 0 \\ 0 & 1 & 0 & T_s \\ 0 & 0 & 1 & 0 \\ 0 & 0 & 0 & 1 \end{bmatrix} \qquad (4.4)$$

$$\text{Measurement matrix, } C = \begin{bmatrix} 1 & 0 & 0 & 0 \\ 0 & 1 & 0 & 0 \end{bmatrix} \qquad (4.5)$$

The two main processes followed in Kalman filtering are prediction and correction. The two-state equations (Anon 2017) governing the motion of the object are:

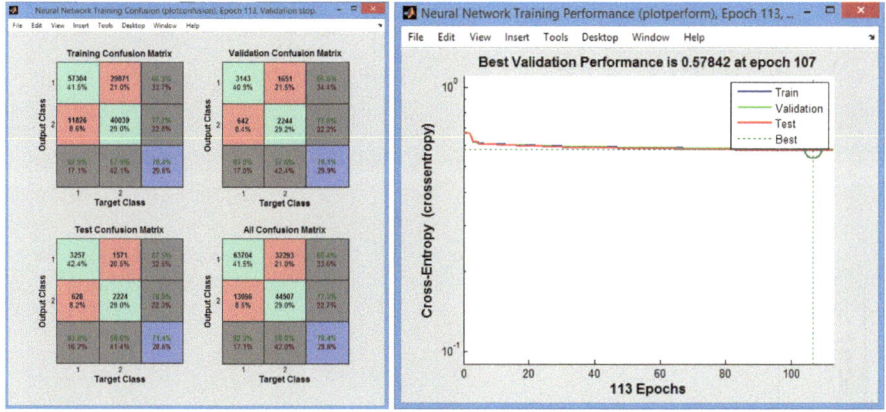

Fig. 4.29 Confusion matrix and performance plot in Subject 2 delta frequency range (figure captured during experimental sessions)

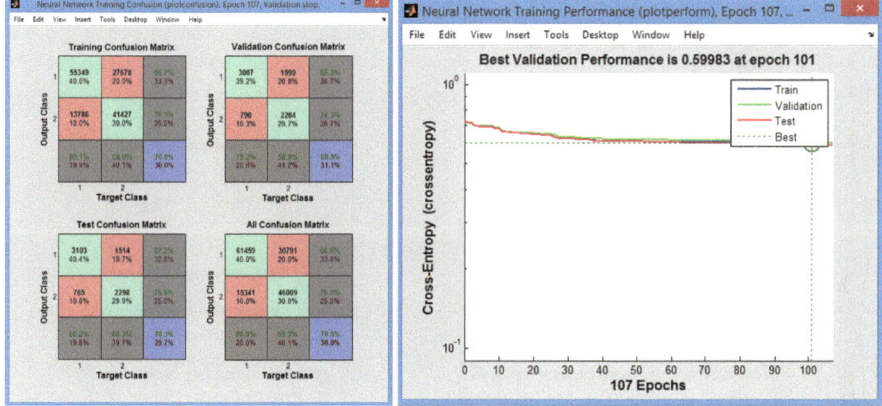

Fig. 4.30 Confusion matrix and performance plot in Subject 2 theta frequency range (figure captured during experimental sessions)

$$\bar{x}_t = A x_{t-1} + B u_t \qquad (4.6)$$

$$\bar{z}_t = C \bar{x}_t + E_Z \qquad (4.7)$$

Figure 4.32 depicts the full recursive procedure followed by the Kalman filter. Prediction part of the filter solves the state Eqs. 4.6 and 4.8 describing the model at the time, $t + 1$. Here, x is the state vector and z is the measurement vector. After a step of prediction, the states are projected to the next step where correction of the error covariance is done. The following set of equations (Anon 2017) is used for minimization of error covariance.

$$\bar{E}_t = A E_{t-1} A^T + E_t \qquad (4.8)$$

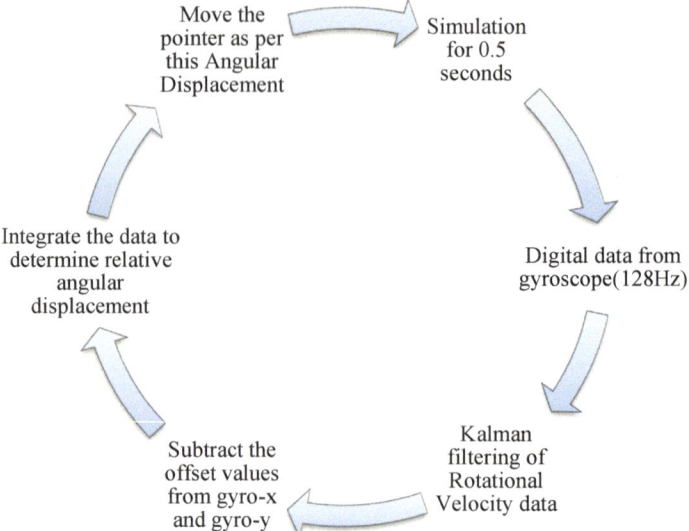

Fig. 4.31 Flowchart for the method of implementation of mouse emulator (figure generated by the authors)

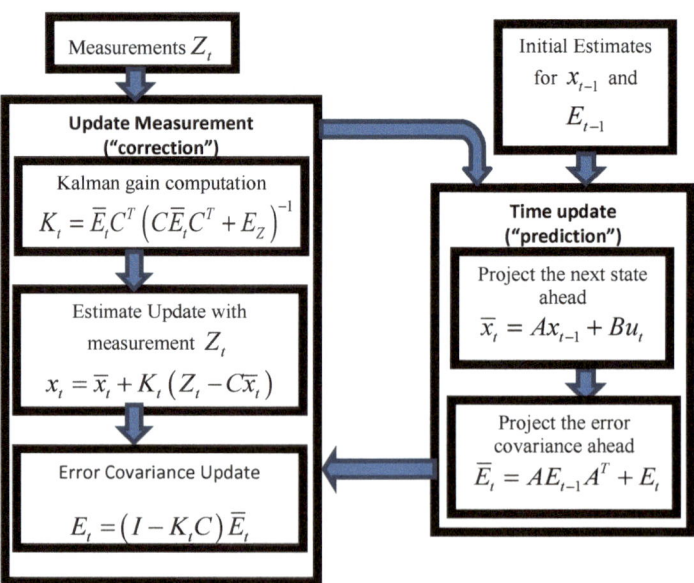

Fig. 4.32 Flowchart for implementation of Kalman filter (figure generated by the authors; equations taken from Anon 2017)

$\bar{E}_t$ denotes the estimated error covariance matrix generated in the step of prediction which follows the abovementioned equation. The next step, initializing the process of "Correction", is to calculate the Kalman gain, K_t using Eq. 4.9. E_Z, which denotes the covariance, when has a high value, leads to a less informative data and hence, a smaller K_t. In other words, the larger value of state covariance gives a more trustworthy value of measurement data and thus a larger value of K_t. Once the Kalman gain is calculated, the next state of the system can be calculated using Eq. 4.10, where the Kalman gain depicts the importance of the incoming measurement data.

$$K_t = \bar{E}_t C^T \left(C \bar{E}_t C^T + E_Z \right)^{-1} \quad \text{(Anon 2017)} \tag{4.9}$$

$$x_t = \bar{x}_t + K_t (Z_t - C \bar{x}_t) \quad \text{(Anon 2017)} \tag{4.10}$$

Next, the error covariance E_t is evaluated using the previously estimated error covariance, $\bar{E}_t$ and the Kalman gain, K_t. So, $\bar{E}_t$ is the error covariance before an update and E_t is the error covariance related to process noise vector whereas, E_z is the error covariance related to the measurement noise vector.

$$E_t = (I - K_t C)\bar{E}_t \quad \text{(Anon 2017)} \tag{4.11}$$

Figure 4.33 shows how gyroscope data has been improvised using Kalman filtering. The process of filtering is followed by removal of offset value from both GYRO-x and GYRO-y signals, which are 1700 and 1600, respectively.

After this, integration is done in order to find out the relative displacement and hence obtain the final data that can be used for implementation. Angular velocity (deg/s) is given as

$$\dot{\theta} = \frac{d\theta}{dt} \tag{4.12}$$

In continuous and discrete form, respectively, angular displacement (Anon 2017) is given as

$$\theta(t) = \int_0^t \dot{\theta}(t) dt \approx \sum_0^t \dot{\theta}(t) T_s \tag{4.13}$$

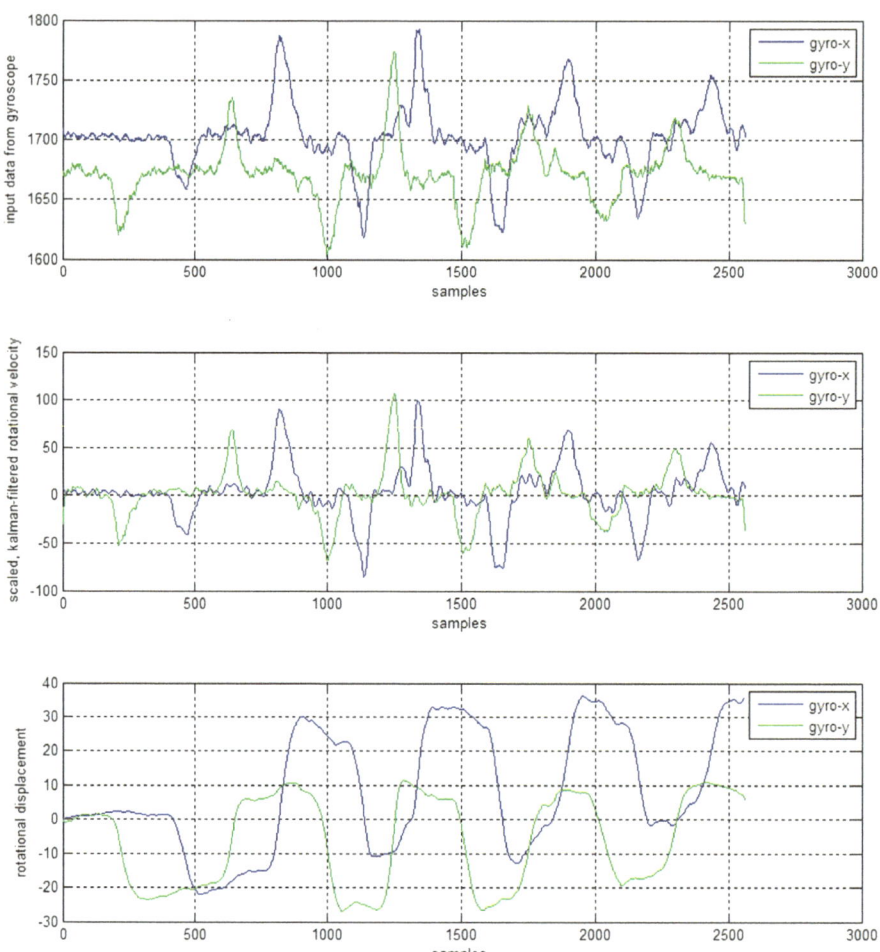

Fig. 4.33 Step-by-step plots of digital data (figure captured during experimental sessions)

4.5   Implementation of BCI Controlling Robot (Robot 1 and 2)

4.5.1   Robot 1 (Fire Bird V ATMEGA2560) Specifications and Implementation of "Control Using BCI"

A graphical user interface designed in MATLAB is used to drive the Fire Bird V-BOT (Fig. 4.34) in all its possible directions. Technical hardware and software specifications have been provided in Table 4.3.

Table 4.3 Robot 1 full specifications (Nex-robotics.com 2017)

	Component	Specifications
Microcontroller	Atmel ATMEGA2560	Master microcontroller
	Atmel ATMEGA8	Slave microcontroller
Sensors	Three white line sensors	Extendable to 7
	Five sharp IR range sensors	GP2D12
	Eight IR proximity sensors	Analog behavior
	Two position encoders	Extendable to 4
	Battery voltage sensing	–
	Current sensing	Optimal
Indicators	LCD	2 × 16 characters
	LEDs (indicators)	–
	Buzzer	–
Control	Autonomous control	
	PC as master and robot as slave	Wired or wireless mode
Communication	Wireless ZigBee Communication	2.4 GHz
	Wired serial communication	RS232
	Infrared communication	Simplex, remote to robot
Dimensions	Diameter	16 cm
	Height	10 cm
	Weight	1300 g
Power	Nickel metal hydride battery pack along with auxiliary power	9.6 V, 2100 mAh
	Life	2 h while motors are operational 75% of the time
Locomotion	Two DC geared motors with a caster wheel in the front	24 cm/s, 51 mm diameter
	Position encoder	30 pulses per revolution
	Position encoder resolution	5.44 mm

4.5.1.1 Interfacing with the PC Through MATLAB

Integrated development environments (IDEs) are a necessary part of programming for AVR microcontrollers. Many of them are available on the internet out of which, some work wholly only for a month or so. The free IDE, AVR Studio from ATMEL uses WIN AVR as an open-source C compiler at the back end. It also has built-in In-Circuit Emulator and an AVR instruction set simulator. A program can be written, compiled, and debugged in this software and then loaded onto the robot using an in-system programmer (ISP). It also supports included AVR Assembler and any external AVR GCC compiler in a complete IDE environment. The two main advantages of AVR Studio can be listed as follows:

Fig. 4.34 FIRE BIRD V
(robot 1) for BCI-controlled
robot application 1 (figure
captured during
experimental sessions,
Nex-robotics.com 2017)

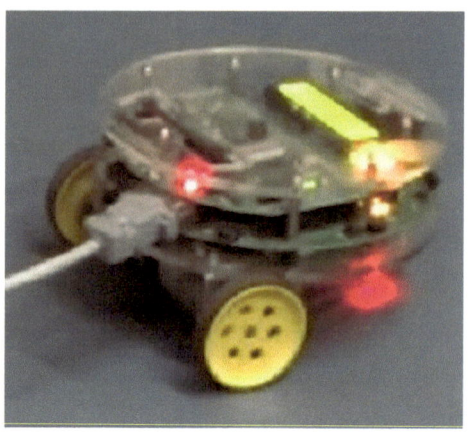

The single application window can be sued to debug and edit also enabled with faster error tracking. Breakpoints are saved and restored between sessions, even if codes are edited.

After opening AVR Studio, a new project can be opened selecting "New Project". The project type is to be chosen as "AVR GCC" and any name can be given. Thus, all the files can be created in this way inside the new folder. The location of the folder can be chosen as per wish in the location window. After this, the debugging platform and device are to be selected as "AVR Simulator" and "ATMEGA2560", respectively. Another important aspect to be noted is the selection of Crystal frequency which is 11.0592 MHz in our case. Optimization level is set at "-O0". "Optimization" option defines the optimization level for all files. Higher optimization levels will produce code that is harder to debug. Stack variables may change location, or be optimized away, and source level debugging may "skip" statements because they too have been optimized away. "-O0" stands for no optimization, that is, the same as not specifying any optimization.

Figure 4.36 shows the pin configuration of the motor driver L293D. There are four inputs here where input 1 is connected to pin 2, input 2 is connected to pin 7, input 3 is connected to pin 10, and input 4 is connected to pin 15. Port A of the microcontroller ATMEGA 2560 which has four pins (PA0, PA1, PA2, and PA3) connects to the input pins of the L293D. Figure 4.35 shows the interfacing between the microcontroller ATMEGA 2560 and DIL-16. Figure 4.37 shows the positioning of the DC geared motors and posiiton encoders in the robot. Now the pin configurations for different directions of motion are found out from the following truth Tables 4.4, 4.5 and 4.6.

After compilation of the program in AVR Studio 8, it provides a "hex" file. This "hex" file needs to be loaded on the robot using in-system programmer (ISP) as mentioned earlier. The ISP programming is done by the Khazama AVR programmer. First, a chip signature is read from the command section. However, an important point to be noted here is, if the work is being done on Windows 8 platform, the digital sig-

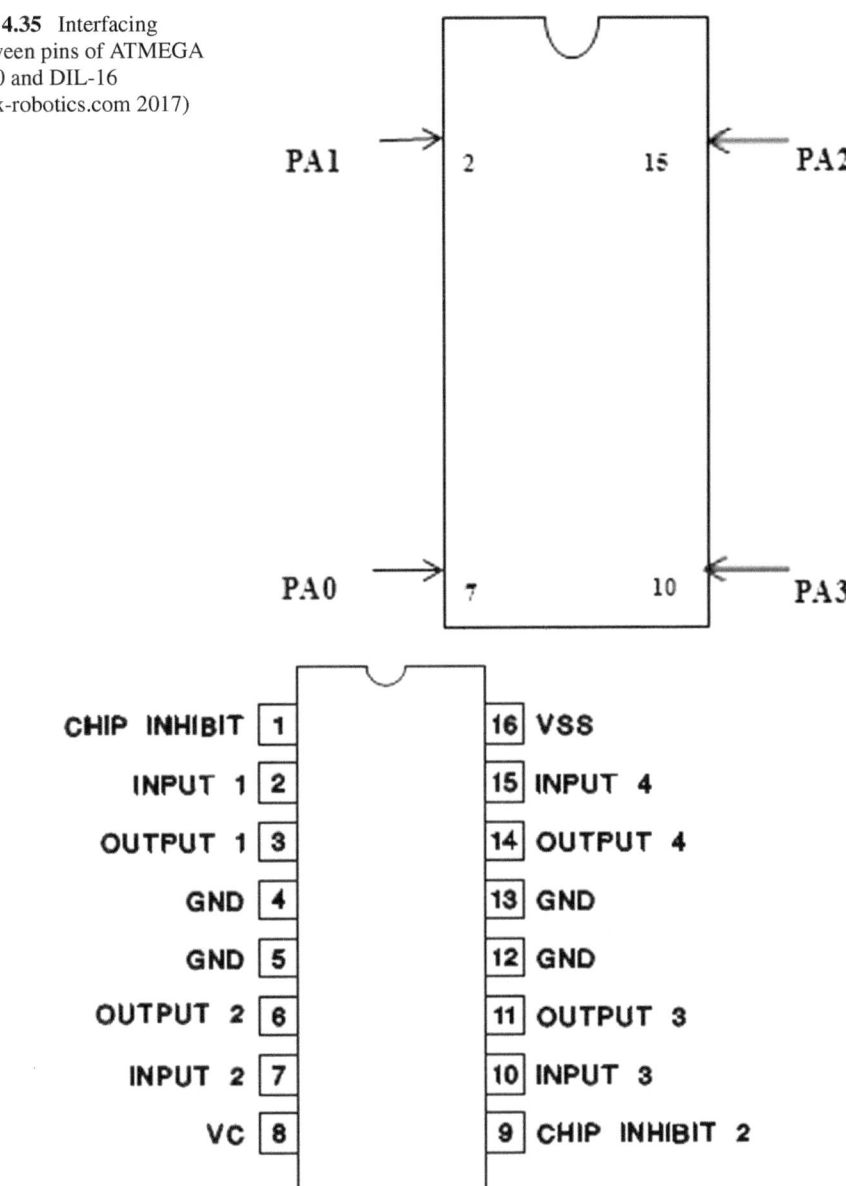

Fig. 4.35 Interfacing between pins of ATMEGA 2560 and DIL-16 (Nex-robotics.com 2017)

Fig. 4.36 Pin configuration of L293D (Nex-robotics.com 2017)

nature verification is to be deactivated as Windows 8 does not allow software without digital signatures to run. The deactivation is done at start-up of the Windows. Afterward, the .hex file generated earlier is loaded to the buffer of Khazama programmer following which, the flash buffer is written to the chip, that is, ATMEGA2560.

Table 4.4 Truth table for motion direction control (Nex-robotics.com 2017)

Direction and pins	Left backward (LB) *PA0*	Left forward (LF) *PA1*	Right forward (RF) *PA2*	Right backward (RB) *PA3*
Forward	0	1	1	0
Reverse	1	0	0	1
Right	0	1	0	1
Left	1	0	1	0
Soft right	0	1	0	0
Soft left	0	0	1	0
Soft right 2	0	0	0	1
Soft left 2	1	0	0	0
Hard stop	0	0	0	0
Soft stop	X	X	X	X

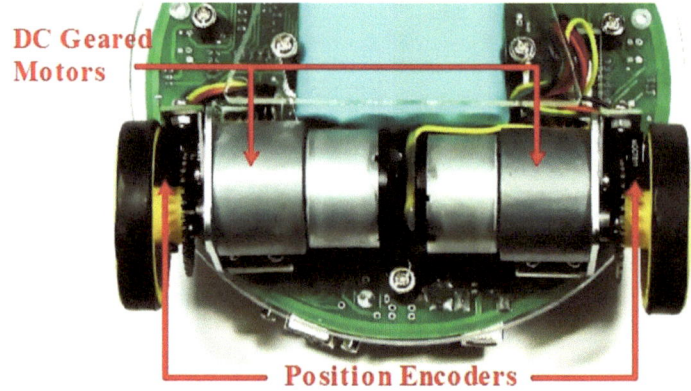

Fig. 4.37 DC geared motors and position encoders in FIRE BIRD V (Nex-robotics.com 2017)

Table 4.5 Pin functions for motion control (Nex-robotics.com 2017)

ATMEGA2560 Microcontroller pin	Function
PA0	Left motor direction control
PA1	Left motor direction control
PA2	Right motor direction control
PA3	Right motor direction control

This will burn the program into the chip. For testing of serial communication between PC and robot and getting the appropriate feedback, the *terminal software* can be used. Figure 4.38 shows how the commands are sent to FIRE BIRD V through HyperTerminal.

Table 4.6 Pin functions of ATMEGA2560 for motion direction control and their hexadecimal equivalent (Nex-robotics.com 2017)

Hexadecimal	Port A of ATMEGA2560				Action
	Port A3	Port A2	Port A1	Port A0	
	Right motor backward	Right motor forward	Left motor forward	Left motor backward	
0X06	0	1	1	0	Forward
0X09	1	0	0	1	Backward (reverse)
0X05	0	1	0	1	Left
0X0A	1	0	1	0	Right
0X00	0	0	0	0	Stop (hard stop)

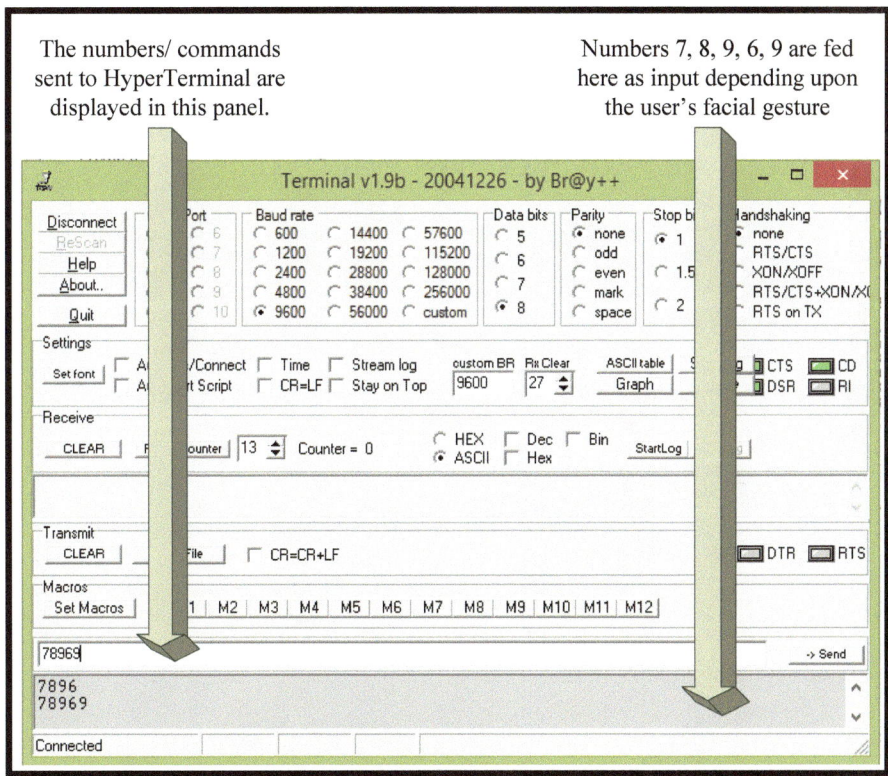

Fig. 4.38 Commands sent to FIRE BIRD V through HyperTerminal (figure captured during experimental sessions)

The robot motions are controlled using BCIs. All possible motions that are included in the Graphical User Interface designed in MATLAB for controlling the Fire Bird V have been mentioned below:

Forward (both the motors move forward),

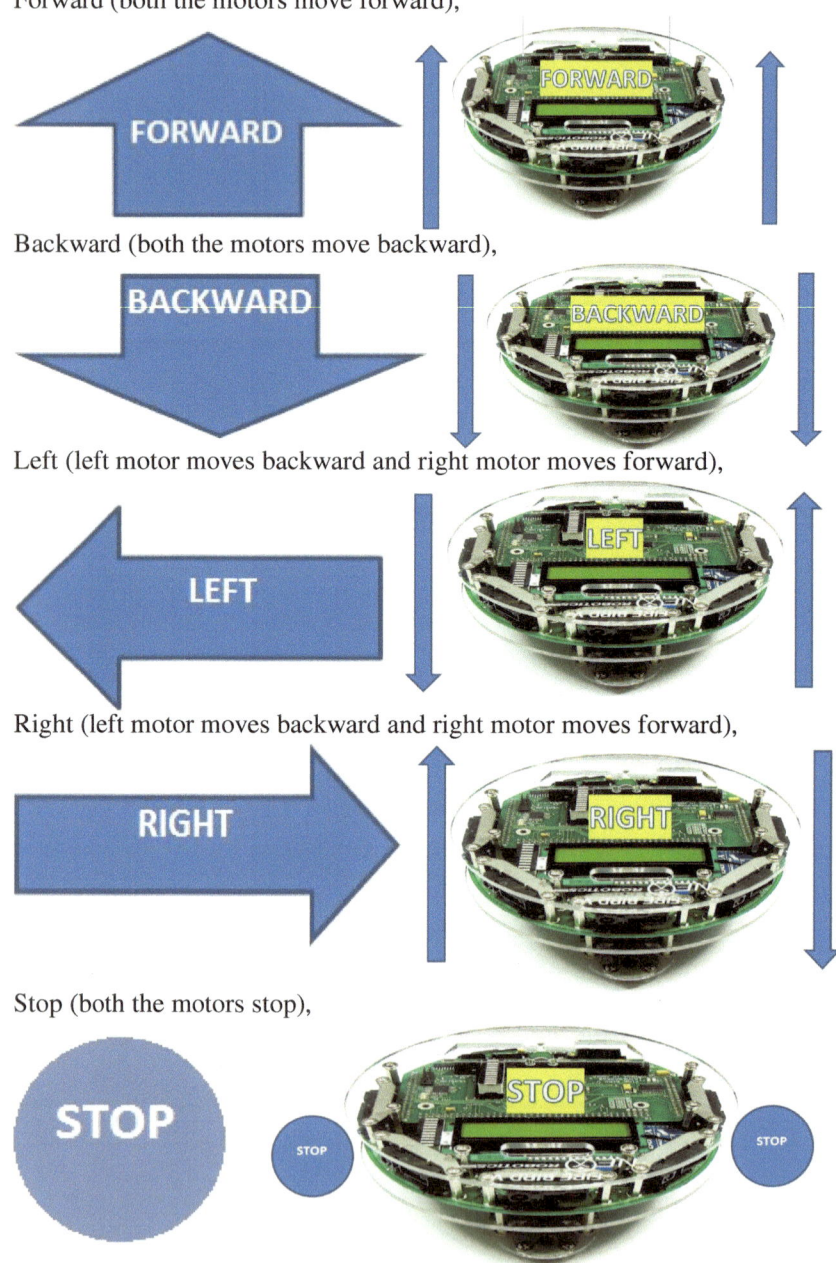

Backward (both the motors move backward),

Left (left motor moves backward and right motor moves forward),

Right (left motor moves backward and right motor moves forward),

Stop (both the motors stop),

Soft left 1 (left motor stops and right motor moves forward),

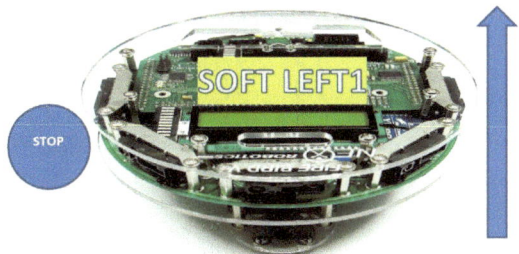

Soft right 1 (left motor moves forward and right motor stops),

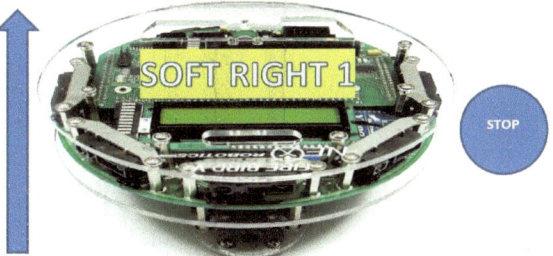

Soft left 2 (left motor moves backward and right motor stops),

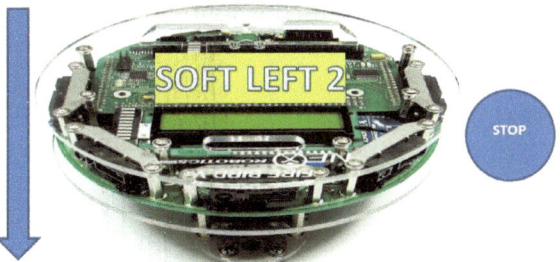

Soft right 2 (left motor stops and right motor moves backward),

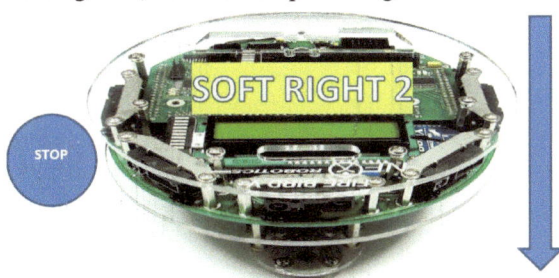

The user communicates with the GUI (depicted in Fig. 4.39) with the help of clicks and cursor movements which have been made possible by acquiring data from the patient's brain through the EPOC headset. This GUI has 9 control buttons (forward, backward, left, right, stop, soft left 1, soft right 1, soft left 2, and soft right 2). When the push button is pressed, the necessary command is passed on to the device FIRE BIRD V through serial communication.

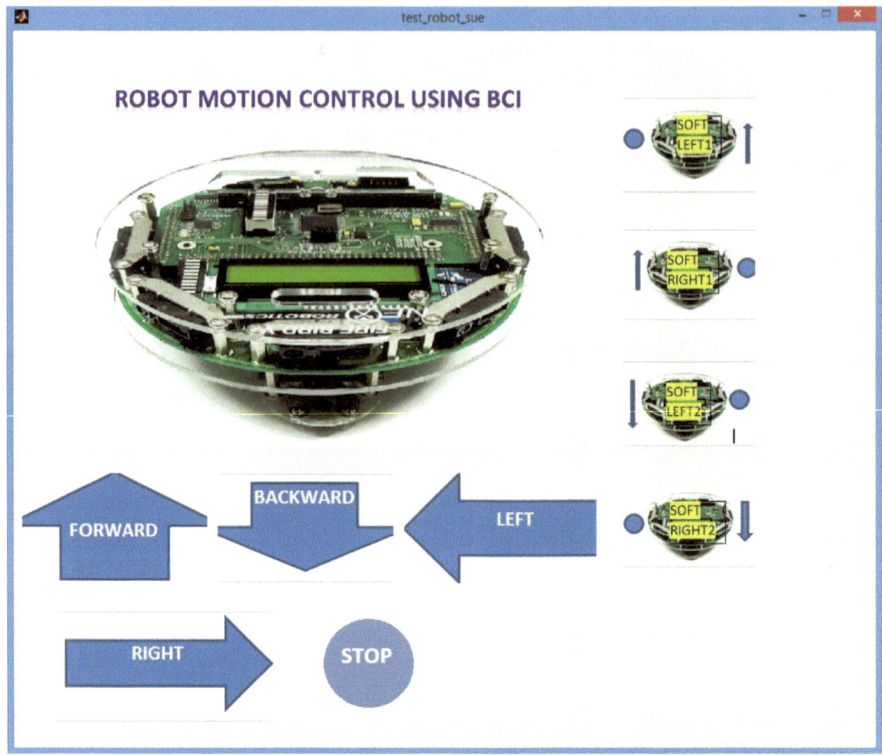

Fig. 4.39 GUI designed for robot 1 in MATLAB (figure generated by the authors)

The above events were generated as per the pin configurations and hex codes in hardware manual. The pins PA0, PA1, PA2, and PA3 of ATMEGA 2560 micro-controller chip were interfaced with pin 7, pin 2, pin 15, and pin 10 of L293D, respectively. Then the robot motions Forward, Backward, Left, Right, Stop, Soft Left1, Soft Right1, Soft Left2, and Soft Right2 were carried out when the device commands "8", "2", "4", "6", "5", "7", "1", "3", "9" were sent to the robot through serial communication. Figure 4.40 shows the flow diagram of an implementation of the robot motion control using BCI.

The patient or the user decides which direction he/she wants to go to through the MATLAB GUI and clicks the respective button in the GUI as per the desired direction.

4.5.2 Robot 2 (Arduino-Based Free-Wheeling Robot) Specifications and Implementation of "Robot Control Using BCI"

Graphical User Interface in MATLAB was designed for driving the robot in any desired direction and in different motions. The robot 2 is based on Freeduino MEGA 2560 board (Fig. 4.41) containing ATmega 2560 microcontroller. The overall hardware specifications have been given below in Table 4.7:

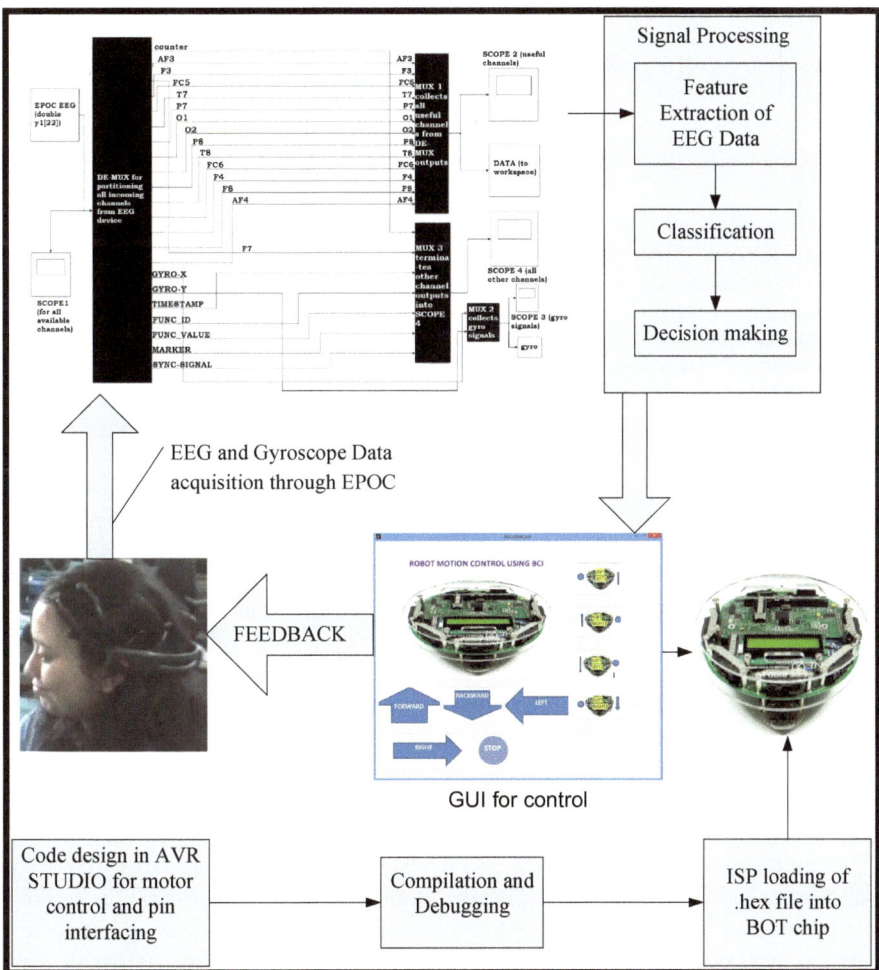

Fig. 4.40 Implementation of robot 1 control through BCI—flow diagram (figure generated by the authors)

Table 4.7 Hardware specifications (Robot 2; Table generated by the authors)

	Component	Specifications
Hardware	Board	Freeduino Mega 2560
	Microcontroller	ATmega 2560
	BOT Chassis	High Strength PVC alloy Unbreakable body
	Wheels (4)	Tracked wheel with 10 cm diameter
	Motor (4)	300 rpm, 30 kg cm DC geared motor
	Motor driver	20 A dual DC motor driver
	Battery	Lithium polymer 3 cell, 11.1 V, 5000 mAh
Software	MATLAB	2013b
	Arduino I/O package for MATLAB	–
	Arduino	Version 1.0.5-r2

Fig. 4.41 Robot 2
Arduino-based autonomous
robot with high powered
speed controllable wheels
(image taken from laboratory
experiments)

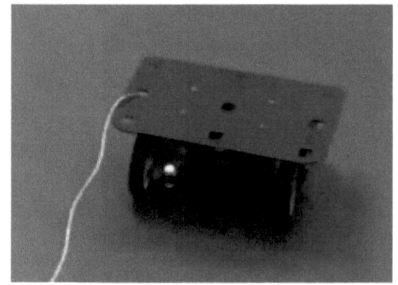

The graphical user interface can be used to convert the facial expressions into real-time commands to be sent to the robot. The process starts with the BCI system converting signals from the patient into mouse click of the computer and then, the graphical user interface converts BCIs output signals into robotic commands in the Arduino board. The GUI also provides feedback to the user in the form of variable images whenever a command is sent to the robot through Arduino board. In this way, the user can teach himself/herself to use the GUI for the desired movements in the robot.

Arduino board has been interfaced with MATLAB software in order to move the robot in its possible directions. Arduino is an open-source electronics prototyping platform based on flexible, easy-to-use hardware and software. It is intended for artists, designers, hobbyists, and anyone interested in creating Interactive objects or environments. (Arduino.cc 2017) Arduino MEGA 2560 is a board with Freeduino MEGA 2560 microcontroller which directly receives serial data from the computer to get delivered to the robot.

The commands generated by MATLAB GUI are sent to the Arduino board which is connected through a USB cable. (Arduino.cc 2017) The Arduino board has 16 analog pins and 54 digital pins out of which 14 provide PWM output. Since the speed of the robot is needed to be controllable, the PWM pins are used.

The board uses Atmega8U2 as its USB to Serial converter. The pins 46, 47, 38, and 36 are, respectively, used to control the directions and braking of left and right motors, which come to the category of digital pins. Pins 3 and 4 are PWM pins used to control the speed of revolution of the robot wheels.

The Arduino MEGA 2560 board was first programmed with Arduino software (sketch) in order to make it capable of receiving and interpreting data successfully and then it is interfaced with the robot and computer to send motion signals and move the robot in any desired motion.

The Arduino digital pins are to be configured as either input or output pins. By default, they are programmed as input pins. The pin.Mode (pin, Mode) command can be used to configure the digital pins. Here, "pin" denotes the pin number to be configured and "Mode" is the desired mode, which can be either "input" or "output".

4.5.2.1 How to Set up an Arduino

The required components are the board and a cable to link plug A and B. By this, the connection between the PC and the board is made. Next, the board is connected to the PC. COM port (Arduino, by default, gets access to one of the serial ports on the PC which are commonly known as the COM ports. Here COM4 is used). The integrated development environment (IDE) software called Arduino is downloaded. Compilation and verification of the sketch are done to initialize serial communication between MATLAB and Arduino board into this software and then this sketch is loaded into the board.

In serial port communication, information gets transferred at the rate of 1 bit at a time. Arduino IO Package allows communicating with an Arduino Uno or MEGA 2560 over a serial port through MATLAB software. It can be obtained as a support package from MATLAB. It comprises of a MATLAB API which is run on the host computer and a server program that runs on the Arduino. When operated altogether, the software allows accessing Arduino analog I/O, digital I/O, operate servo motors, read encoders, and even handling dc and stepper motors using the Adafruit Motor shield, all by using MATLAB command lines. Initialization of the Arduino board is done by a command as follows (Sets COM4 as the COM port for interfacing):

$$a = arduino(COM4)$$

For the patient to gain proper control over the designed system, he/she needs to be trained with patience. After this process, the user is allowed to access the GUI. The elements included in the GUI have been explained in detail in the following section.

4.5.2.2   Possible robot motions

		Forward motion: Clicking this button will make the robot move in a forward direction. That is, both sides, the motors move in a forward direction.
		Moving left: Clicking this button will make the robot take a left turn. The right motors move forward and left motors move backward.
		Moving softleft_1: Clicking this button will make the robot take a very soft left turn. The left motors do not move and the right motors move in a forward direction.
		Moving softleft_2: Clicking this button makes robot take another type of a very soft left turn. The right motors are braked (stopped) and left motors are moved backward.
		Stopping robot : Clicking this will be braking the robot to halt. It will stop all the motors.
		Moving softright_1: Clicking this pushbutton will make the robot take a very soft right turn marked by right motor braked (stopped) and left motor moving in the forward direction.

	Forward in High Speed: This attribute is to move the robot at a comparatively higher speed as normal motion. Both side motors move in the same direction.
	Moving right: Clicking this button makes the robot take a sharp right turn marked by left motor moving in the forward direction and right motors in a backward direction.
	Moving softright_2: Clicking this button will make the robot take a soft right turn with the right motor moving in a backward direction and left motor stopped.
	Backward motion: Clicking this button will make the robot move backward, that is, both left and right motors will move in the backward direction.

The patient must decide in which direction he has to move and click the button accordingly with the help of his/her facial expression generated EEG signal. The full working diagram has been shown in the next flowchart (Fig. 4.42).

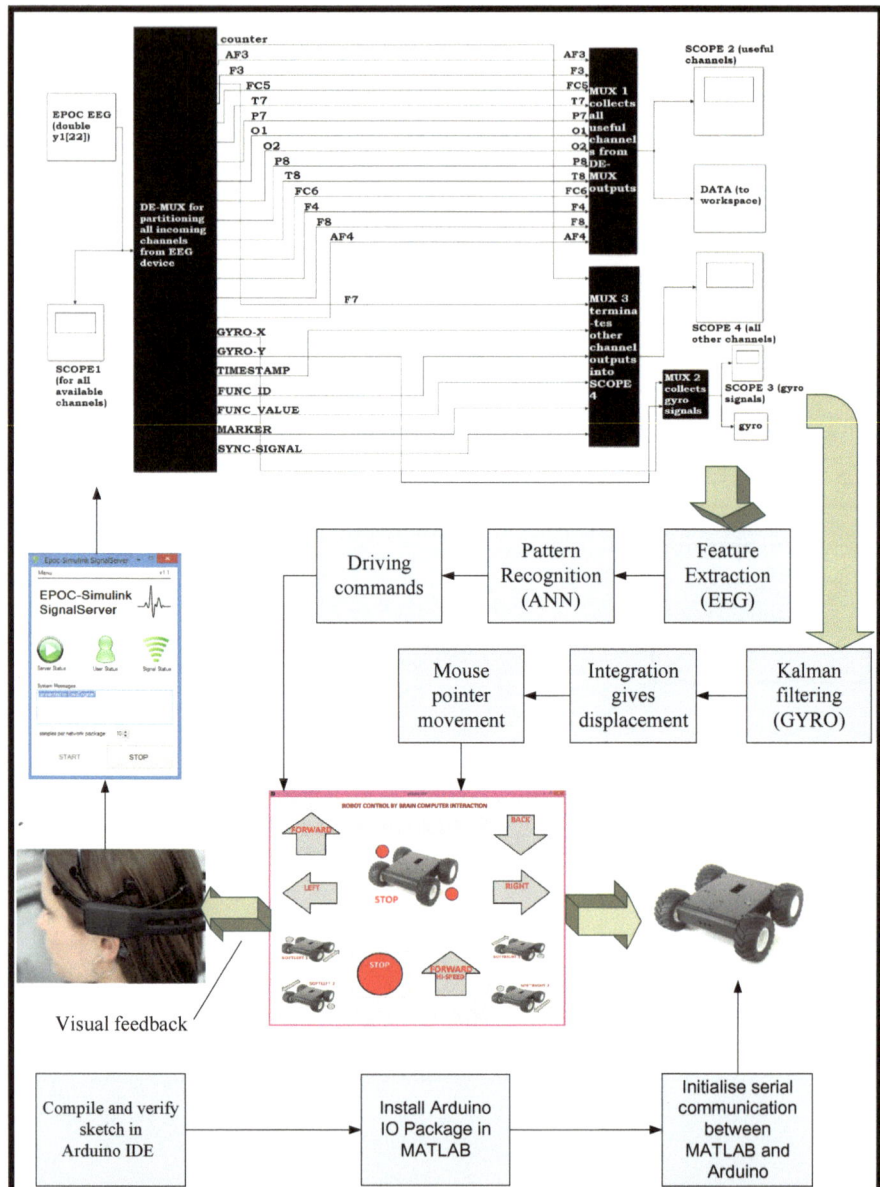

Fig. 4.42   Implementation of robot 2 controlled by BCI (figure generated by the authors)

References

Anon. 2017. *Student Dave's Tutorials* [online]. Available at: http://studentdavestutorials.weebly.com/.

Arduino.cc. 2017. *Arduino—Home* [online]. Available at: https://www.arduino.cc/.

Haar, A. 1911. Zur theorie der orthogonalen funktionensysteme. *Mathematische Annalen* 71 (1): 38–53.

McFarland, D.J., and Wolpaw, J.R. 2008. Brain-computer interface operation of robotic and prosthetic devices. *Computer* 41(10).

Nex-robotics.com. 2017. *Fire Bird V ATMEGA2560 robotic research platform—Nex robotics* [online]. Available at: http://www.nex-robotics.com/products/fire-bird-v-robots/fire-bird-v-atmega2560-robotic-research-platform.html.

Ra.cs.uni-tuebingen.de. 2017. *Scaled conjugate gradient (SCG)* [online]. Available at: http://www.ra.cs.uni-tuebingen.de/SNNS/UserManual/node241.html.

Wold, S., K. Esbensen, and P. Geladi. 1987. Principal component analysis. *Chemometrics and Intelligent Laboratory Systems* 2 (1–3): 37–52.

Chapter 5
Results and Conclusion

Abstract This section summarizes the quantitative results of the experiments carried out during the assembling of the final prototype. The major participant algorithm in the system is the neural network that classifies the electroencephalographic signals received from the user's brain and makes the decision of what was intended through the process. Therefore, the numerical results in this section include the classification accuracies obtained by using various classes of the electroencephalographic signals (based on frequency bands). In the second phase of the results, support vector machine has been used to measure accuracies for multiple subjects while performing various operations. This section also summarizes the same. Five types of operations were directly considered for classification using support vector machine. Classification accuracies obtained were not as good as a neural network, but acceptable. Based on the results in this section, the end algorithm was obtained which gave the highest accuracies in overall performance. Future work will include betterment of the algorithms and inclusion of a higher number of subjects for data collection and corroboration.

5.1 Classification Results—1

In the first phase of work, a self-algorithm for the control of a secondary device through EEG signals was designed in offline mode. It gave good results and high rates of accuracy in classification. Following tables show the accuracies of classification of offline data in the three subjects considering all four possible gestures (Tables 5.1, 5.2, 5.3, 5.4, 5.5, 5.6, 5.7).

It can be seen that the highest percentage of accuracies (highlighted) can be obtained in the Beta ranges of frequencies in all the three subjects. We obtain very high classification accuracies in the offline mode of classification of EEG data. However, the real-time processing of the same data differs to some extent. The significance of high accuracy in Beta frequency range has been explained in the later part of this section. In the second part of our work, the already-developed algorithm is used as a real-time algorithm. The main difference between the two implementations is that,

© The Author(s), under exclusive license to Springer Nature Singapore Pte Ltd. 2019   105
S. Das et al., *Real-Time BCI System Design to Control Arduino Based Speed Controllable Robot Using EEG*, SpringerBriefs in Computational Intelligence,
https://doi.org/10.1007/978-981-13-3098-8_5

Table 5.1 Offline classification accuracy results of subject 1

DWT coefficient	Classification accuracy using neural network after PCA (%)				
	Blink	Neutral	Smile	Raise brow	Overall accuracy
A4 (Delta)	97.0	99.1	97.7	97.3	97.8
D4 (Theta)	96.6	97.6	88.7	94.6	94.6
D3 (Alpha)	89.2	84.3	94.2	93.5	90.0
D2 (Beta)	100	98.3	99.7	97.3	**98.8**
D1 (Gamma)	51.8	39.9	80.7	45.2	53.4

Table 5.2 Offline classification accuracy results of subject 2

DWT coefficient	Classification accuracy using neural network after PCA (%)				
	Blink	Neutral	Smile	Raise brow	Overall accuracy
A4 (Delta)	93.9	89.3	81.0	89.3	88.2
D4 (Theta)	81.7	84.5	77.9	82.4	81.6
D3 (Alpha)	30.7	84.2	97.9	94.8	68.4
D2 (Beta)	95.4	95.4	97.9	94.8	**94.9**
D1 (Gamma)	46.1	37.3	61.3	55.0	50.9

Table 5.3 Offline classification accuracy results of subject 3

DWT coefficient	Classification accuracy using neural network after PCA (%)				
	Blink	Neutral	Smile	Raise brow	Overall accuracy
A4 (Delta)	96.6	98.1	96.0	89.8	95.0
D4 (Theta)	95.7	82.9	86.9	88.3	88.5
D3 (Alpha)	81.5	83.8	89.0	84.4	84.5
D2 (Beta)	97.5	98.5	97.1	92.3	**96.3**
D1 (Gamma)	96.7	72.9	84.8	70.0	81.3

Table 5.4 Real-time classification accuracies in subject 1

DWT coefficient	Classification accuracy of combination under consideration (%)	
	Smile and neutral	Raise brow and neutral
A4 (Delta)	87.6	82.5
D4 (Theta)	76.3	77.8
D3 (Alpha)	84.8	78.9
D2 (Beta)	**91.9**	**89.8**
D1 (Gamma)	90.8	88.2

Table 5.5 Real-time classification accuracies in subject 2

DWT Coefficient	Classification accuracy of combination under consideration (%)	
	Smile and neutral	Raise brow and neutral
A4 (Delta)	70.4	75.6
D4 (Theta)	70.0	70.8
D3 (Alpha)	73.4	72.6
D2 (Beta)	**81.2**	79.8
D1 (Gamma)	81.0	**80.8**

Table 5.6 Actions performed while data collection phase - 2

Types of action	Duration (s)
Forward	60.0
Backward	60.0
Left	10.0
Right	10.0
Neutral	10.0

Table 5.7 Real-time classification accuracies in subjects

Subject	Accuracy (%)
Subject 1	81.5078
Subject 2	78.8274
Subject 3	82.3370
Subject 4	81.9945
Subject 5	80.8542
Subject 6	80.9384
Subject 7	81.7672

when it is done in real time, a set of 64 samples of EEG data are considered at a time for applying the algorithm. Thus, the algorithm is implemented repeatedly every time a set of 64 samples of EEG are received at the acquisition end.

Implementation of the previously developed algorithm has been done in real time in the second phase and successful outcomes have been acquired. Two types of combinations have been taken under consideration, namely, "smile and neutral" and "raise brow and neutral" for classification-based interaction with MATLAB GUI. Blink gesture has not been considered because, whenever the user is concentrating on the GUI on the computer, his neutral state will also include blinks in it. This situation has been taken into consideration while recording the neutral data by making the subject keep open his/her eyes. The following tabular representations depict the various accuracies while training the various data in various ranges of frequencies. Highlighted data show the ones with the highest accuracies.

Highest accuracies have always been found in the beta and gamma ranges of frequencies. The classification has been done using the neural network with 10 hidden neurons and scaled conjugate gradient in the training algorithm. The accuracies given in the above tables are the classification accuracy of the training data which is 90% of the total data samples available from the database. The above observations can be used to conclude that the marked blocks give the highest accuracies which include Beta and Gamma ranges of frequencies. This completely makes sense because the same frequency ranges mark the brain's involvement in some focused or concentration-based activity, which is true when the user is trying to drive the moving robot through the GUI.

As shown in the tabular observations, two types of facial gesture combinations have been used to train the classification data. This gives us a futuristic idea on which combination is a more feasible one. This has been shown that the combination of smile and neutral gestures stands better that the combination of raise brow and neutral. Accuracies can also be observed to be higher in the case of smile and neutral. Apart from that, an important disadvantage of using raise brow and neutral as a combination is that, raising brows at times affects the gyroscope data sent to the working system. This gives unwanted changes in the mouse pointer making it problematic for the user to operate the GUI.

Another important observation on the robots used in our work is that the Arduino-based robot appears to provide more power and control to the user as compared to the FIRE BIRDV-robot. Apart from that, the Arduino robot has the abilities to be controlled in terms of its speed providing more powerful wheels.

A conclusion worth mentioning here is that the mouse clicks produced by using the developed algorithm in real time are fast and precise in nature and can be readily used for operating any GUI implemented in MATLAB or any other platform. In the case of the gyroscope, the involvement of Kalman filter was very important for removal of unwanted jitter from the signals obtained from the gyroscope. This has resulted in a steady motion of the pointer produced by the gyroscope data.

5.2 Classification Results—2

In the second phase of work, a different set of activities were asked to be performed by seven other subjects, as listed below, using the same headset, that is, EmotivEpoc+.

The data collected from seven subjects performing each of the above-mentioned action were collected in EEG format (from 14 electrodes) and then PCA was applied to this data. PCA was applied using **libpca**, a C++ library for Linux and MacOSX. The first four components of the PCA data were used in the next level. The next step was to classify the data using SVM. The predicted classes obtained after classification were compared with the original classes to verify the accuracies, by using **libsvm.** The respective accuracies obtained for the various subjects are listed below.

SVM gives acceptable results of classification of EEG signals. Three types of kernels were considered before obtaining the final results—simple, gaussian, and RBF, and RBF was found to give the best results, which are summarized in the table above.

5.3 Future Scope

An important advantage is that this product can be advanced by introducing obstacle avoidance algorithms in the Arduino robot by interfacing with hi-speed sensors such as KINECT. It can also be advanced by introducing more gestures and providing the user with easier control over the application.

Other possible applications include the replacement of the robots already used by other devices such as robotic arms for providing a *helping hand* to immovable patients; wheelchair by which a user can move to any location by EEG-controlled signals.